NEURODEGENERATIVE DISEASES - LABORATORY AND CLINICAL RESEARCH

HUNTINGTON'S DISEASE

SYMPTOMS, RISK FACTORS AND PROGNOSIS

NEURODEGENERATIVE DISEASES - LABORATORY AND CLINICAL RESEARCH

Additional books in this series can be found on Nova's website under the Series tab.

Additional E-books in this series can be found on Nova's website under the E-book tab.

NEURODEGENERATIVE DISEASES - LABORATORY AND CLINICAL RESEARCH

HUNTINGTON'S DISEASE

SYMPTOMS, RISK FACTORS AND PROGNOSIS

KEVIN GUILLORY
AND
ALEX M. CARRASCO
EDITORS

New York

For permission to use material from this book please contact us:
Telephone 631-231-7269; Fax 631-231-8175
Web Site: http://www.novapublishers.com

Library of Congress Cataloging-in-Publication Data

ISBN: 978-1-62808-316-3

Published by Nova Science Publishers, Inc. † New York

Contents

Preface

Huntington's disease (HD) is a progressive, neurodegenerative genetic disorder characterized by motor dysfunctions, cognitive decline, and psychiatric symptoms. In this book, the authors discuss the symptoms, risk factors and prognosis in Huntington's disease. Topics include the pathogenic mechanisms by which the expanded polyglutamine huntingtin causes neuronal dysfunction and death and the potential therapeutic strategies recently developed for this incurable disorder; the role of brain-derived neurotrophic factor in Huntington's disease; and the legal ramifications in relation to evolving impairments of capacity which can have an outcome in terms of involuntary status as mental health patients, testamentary capacity and the need for guardianship and administration orders.

Chapter I – Huntington’s disease (HD) is a progressive, neurodegenerative disorder characterized by motor dysfunction, cognitive decline, and psychiatric symptoms. Different from the most common forms of other neurodegenerative disorders, such as Parkinson’s disease and Alzheimer’s disease, HD is a monogenic, fully penetrant genetic disorder caused by expansions of a CAG trinucleotide repeat, encoding a polyglutamine tract, in the *huntingtin* gene. HD belongs to the family of polyglutamine diseases, which includes at least eight other neurodegenerative disorders. Polyglutamine diseases share several genetic features and pathogenetic mechanisms leading to neurodegeneration. Among all the polyglutamine diseases, Huntington’s disease is the most common disease. Although the HD causative gene was discovered almost 20 years ago, the mechanism through which expansion of the polyglutamine tract in huntingtin causes neuronal dysfunction and death remains elusive. Expansion of polyglutamine tract confers a gain of toxic function to mutant huntingtin. Here, the authors summarize the pathogenic mechanisms by which the expanded polyglutamine huntingtin causes neuronal dysfunction and death and the potential therapeutic strategies recently developed for this incurable disorder.

Chapter II – Huntington's disease (HD) is the most common polyglutamine neurodegenerative disorder and is caused by a mutation of an unstable expansion of CAG repeats within the coding region of the *HD* gene, which expresses the protein huntingtin. Although the abnormal protein is ubiquitously expressed throughout the organism, cell degeneration occurs mainly in the brain, particularly in the striatum and cortex. The first symptoms usually appear in mid-life and include cognitive deficits and motor disturbances associated with the loss of voluntary movement coordination, which progress over time. The disease is invariably fatal and there is currently no cure for affected individuals. Although the function of normal huntingtin is still under debate, it is now known that this protein can promote the expression of the neurotrophin brain-derived neurotrophic factor (BDNF), as well as its vesicular transport along the microtubules. On the other hand, mutant huntingtin appears to impair both the neuronal expression and transport of this neurotrophic factor, thus contributing to a loss of neurotrophic support in the HD brain. In agreement with this idea, BDNF has been repeatedly shown to be down regulated both in HD patients as well as transgenic and knock-in HD mouse models. In this chapter the authors review the evidence implicating this important neurotrophic factor in the neuropathology of HD and discuss how increasing trophic support in the HD brain might be of potential clinical relevance for the treatment of this devastating neurodegenerative disorder.

Chapter III – Huntington's disease (HD) has serious and disabling mental as well as physical effects, in particular symptoms of depression, impulsivity and paranoia. Such symptoms impact upon those who have HD, those with the potential to inherit it, and those who care for and are close to persons with HD. The symptoms can have many legal ramifications, including in relation to evolving impairments of capacity which can have an outcome in terms of involuntary status as mental health patients, testamentary capacity and the need for guardianship and administration orders. The evolving disease can have effects upon fitness for parenting, obligations to pay spousal and child maintenance, and the quantum of compensation from a tortious incident to which a person is entitled. It can have repercussions for criminal liability and culpability. This chapter reviews case law from a number of countries in relation to such matters, noting the broader radiation to relatives and carers of the effects of HD, and reflecting on the need for legal and medical professionals to be aware of the legal consequences of HD so that they can discharge their responsibilities holistically, sensitively and informedly.

In: Huntington's Disease
Editors: K. Guillory, A. M. Carrasco
ISBN: 978-1-62808-316-3

Chapter I

Huntington's Disease: From Disease Pathogenesis to Clinical Perspectives

***Sara Parodi*[1] *and Maria Pennuto*[1*]**

[1]Department of Neuroscience and Brain Technologies, Istituto Italiano di Tecnologia, Genoa, Italy

Abstract

Huntington's disease (HD) is a progressive, neurodegenerative disorder characterized by motor dysfunction, cognitive decline, and psychiatric symptoms. Different from the most common forms of other neurodegenerative disorders, such as Parkinson's disease and Alzheimer's disease, HD is a monogenic, fully penetrant genetic disorder caused by expansions of a CAG trinucleotide repeat, encoding a polyglutamine tract, in the *huntingtin* gene. HD belongs to the family of polyglutamine diseases, which includes at least eight other neurodegenerative disorders. Polyglutamine diseases share several genetic features and pathogenetic mechanisms leading to neurodegeneration. Among all the polyglutamine diseases, Huntington's disease is the most common disease. Although the HD causative gene

* Corresponding author: Maria Pennuto, PhD, Group Leader, Department of Neuroscience and Brain Technologies, Italian Institute of Technology, via Morego 30, Genoa, 16163, Italy, Phone +39 010 71781793, Fax +39 010 71781230, E-mail: maria.pennuto@iit.it.

was discovered almost 20 years ago, the mechanism through which expansion of the polyglutamine tract in huntingtin causes neuronal dysfunction and death remains elusive. Expansion of polyglutamine tract confers a gain of toxic function to mutant huntingtin. Here, we summarize the pathogenic mechanisms by which the expanded polyglutamine huntingtin causes neuronal dysfunction and death and the potential therapeutic strategies recently developed for this incurable disorder.

Clinical Features of Huntington's Disease

Huntington's disease (HD, OMIM 143100) is a neurodegenerative disorder caused by the expansion of a CAG trinucleotide repeat in the coding region of the *interesting transcript 5* (IT-15) gene (1993). HD is inherited in an autosomal dominant fashion. The gene codes for huntingtin, and the mutation results in an elongated polyglutamine (polyQ) tract in the amino-terminus of the protein. HD is characterized by the progressive loss of medium-sized projection spiny neurons in the caudate nucleus and putamen in the striatum. HD is also associated with widespread degeneration in other brain regions, such as cerebral cortex, hippocampus, thalamus, globus pallidus, subthalamic nucleus, substantia nigra, white matter, and cerebellum (Rosas et al., 2005; Rosas et al., 2003; Rosas et al., 2008). The disease is characterized by motor dysfunction, which initiates with chorea, dystonia, and movement incoordination, and that culminates in loss of the ability to move, bradykinesia, and rigidity in the final stages of the disease. These symptoms are associated with impairment of cognitive functions, such as attention, memory, executive function, as well as with psychiatric symptoms, including change in personality, depression, psychosis, and dementia, which often precede the onset of motor symptoms. Other symptoms include body weight loss, muscle atrophy, cardiac dysfunction, testicular atrophy, as well as endocrine abnormalities, which all become particularly evident as disease progresses (Novak and Tabrizi, 2011).

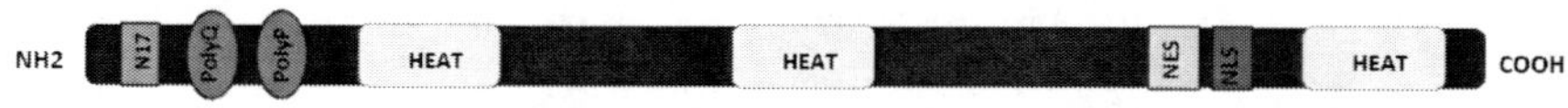

Figure 1. Scheme of htt protein. Full-length htt is composed of 3144 amino acids, with a molecular weight of 350kDa. The amino-terminus of htt contains the highly conserved N17 region and the polyglutamine (polyQ) and polyproline (polyP) tracts. Up to 16 HEAT repeats organized in clusters have been identified in htt. The carboxy-terminus contains a nuclear export signal (NES) and a nuclear localization signal (NLS).

Huntingtin's Structure and Post-Translational Modifications

Normal huntingtin (htt) is composed of 3144 amino acids with a predicted molecular mass of about 350 kDa (Figure 1). The size and mass of htt are variable depending on the number of glutamine residues in the polyQ tract. The polyQ tract in wild type htt ranges from 6 to 35 glutamine residues, and expansion over 36 glutamine causes disease (1993). The polyQ stretch is flanked by two conserved protein domains in vertebrates, the amino-terminal 17-amino-acid sequence (N1-17 domain), and a polyproline region (polyP). The polyP domain modulates the structure of the adjacent polyQ stretch and is a binding site for several htt interacting proteins (Kim et al., 2009; Neveklovska et al., 2012).

On the other hand, the N1-17 domain works as a nuclear export signal (NES) interacting with the nuclear pore protein translocated promoter region (TPR). Expansion of the polyQ tract affects this interaction and leads to the accumulation of mutant htt into the nucleus (Cornett et al., 2005). The N1-17 domain is also required to correctly target htt to various intracellular-membrane-bound organelles, such as the plasma membrane, mitochondria, endosomal/autophagic vescicles, Golgi apparatus, and the endoplasmic reticulum (Atwal et al., 2007; Kegel et al., 2005; Rockabrand et al., 2007). Htt contains multiple HEAT (hungtintin, elongation factor 3, the PR65/A subunit of protein phosphatase 2A and the lipid kinase Tor) repeat sequences. A recent study showed that htt contains 16 HEAT repeats organized in 4 clusters. A HEAT repeat is a degenerate ~50 amino-acid sequence involved in protein-protein interactions (Tartari et al., 2008).

Recent evidence suggests that protein context and post-translational modifications can influence the neurotoxicity of polyQ proteins (Pennuto et al., 2009). Htt undergoes several post-translational modifications, such as phosphorylation, SUMOylation, acetylation, palmitoylation, ubiquitylation, and proteolytic cleavage. Phosphorylation of polyQ-htt at serine 421 by Akt results in decreased formation of nuclear inclusions and reduced toxicity in cultured striatal neurons (Crippa et al., 2010; Humbert et al., 2002) and in an HD rodent model (Pardo et al., 2006). Inhibition of the phosphatase calcineurin (PP2B) increases polyQ-htt phosphorylation at serine 421 and reduces striatal neuronal death (Pardo et al., 2006). Intracellular transport is affected by expansion of the polyQ tract in htt, and this function is restored by phosphorylation at serine 421 (Colin et al., 2008; Zala et al., 2008). To highlight the importance of this modification in HD is the observation that serine 421 phosphorylation is reduced in the cortex and striatum of HD mice (Warby et al., 2005). The 17 amino acids before the polyQ tract also contain phosphorylated sites. IkappaB kinase (IKK) complex phosphorylates serine 13, which triggers the phosphorylation of serine 16 (Thompson et al., 2009). Phosphorylation at these residues increases the degradation of normal htt by targeting the protein to the proteasome and lysosome (Thompson et al., 2009). Mouse models expressing full-length polyQ-htt with serine 13 and 16 substituted by phospho-mimetic aspartate and phospho-defective alanine have been created by Gu and colleagues (Gu et al., 2009). Constitutive phosphorylation at these sites ameliorates the HD phenotype, while the clinical and molecular symptoms of HD are preserved when the serine are mutated to alanine (Gu et al., 2009). The most prevalent amino-terminal modification is the phosphorylation of threonine 3. Aiken and colleagues showed that phospho-defective and phospho-mimetic mutantions at this site can affect the toxicity of polyQ-htt in HD flies (Aiken et al., 2009). CDK5 phosphorylates htt at serines 434, 1181, and 1201 (Anne et al., 2007; Luo et al., 2005). The impact of these phosphorylation events on HD phenotype is different depending on the specific site involved. For instance, phosphorylation at serine 434 reduces htt cleavage by caspases and decreases the toxicity of the expanded polyQ protein. Phosphorylation at serine 1181 and 1201 protects against toxicity, while absence of phosphorylation at the same sites conversely confers toxic properties to the normal protein (Anne et al., 2007; Luo et al., 2005).

The binding of ubiquitin to a protein occurs through an isopeptide bond formed between lysine residues in a target protein and the carboxy-terminal group of ubiquitin. Ubiquitylation controls the stability, function, and intracellular localization of htt, thereby contributing to maintain htt homeostasis in the cells. Htt has been shown to be ubiquitylated at lysines 6, 9, and 15 and to be targeted to the proteasome for degradation (DiFiglia, 1997; Kalchman et al., 1996).

The covalent and reversible attachment of the SUMO (small ubiquitin-related modifier) proteins to the side chain of lysine residues in the target protein is referred to as SUMOylation. In cultured cells, SUMOylation of the N-terminal domain of polyQ-htt stabilizes the protein, reduces its ability to form aggregates, and promotes its ability to repress transcription. In a Drosophila model of HD, SUMOylation of polyQ-htt has been shown to exacerbate neurodegeneration (Steffan et al., 2004).

The covalent binding of an acetyl group to lysine residues is a reversible reaction catalyzed by histone acetyltransferase (HAT) enzymes, and its removal is operated by histone deacetylase (HDAC) enzymes. Recently, five new lysine acetylation sites were identified, including three novel sites K178, K236, K345, and two previously described sites, K9 and K444 (Cong et al., 2011). Increased acetylation at K444 facilitates trafficking of polyQ-htt into autophagosomes, significantly improves clearance of the mutant protein by macroautophagy, and reverses the toxic effects of polyQ-htt in primary striatal and cortical neurons and in a transgenic C. elegans model of HD (Jeong et al., 2009).

Palmitoylation is the reversible covalent attachment of a saturated palmitic fatty acid chain to a cysteine residue of proteins. Htt is palmitoylated at C214 by the palmitoyl transferase hungtintin interacting protein (HIP) 14. Expansion of the polyQ tract reduces the interaction between htt and HIP14 and decreases the amount of palmitoylated polyQ-htt. Importantly, loss of htt palmitoylation exacerbates toxicity, as it results in increased protein aggregation and cell death (Yanai et al., 2006).

Transglutaminases are a family of calcium-activated enzymes that catalyze the acyl transfer reaction between glutamine residues of a protein and lysine residues of another protein, leading to generation of isopeptide bonds that cross-link proteins. The evidence that transglutaminase activity is important in the pathogenesis of HD comes from the observation that ablation of the gene encoding type 2 transglutaminase in HD mice alleviates disease manifestations (Mastroberardino et al., 2002). On the other hand, the overexpression of type 2 tranglutaminase in cultured striatal neurons expressing either wild type or polyQ-htt had the opposite effect on cell survival, suggesting that sensitivity of striatal neurons to transglutaminase activity may depend on cellular context (Ruan et al., 2007).

Different from most of other post-translational modifications, the process of proteolysis is irreversible. Htt was the first protein involved in a neurodegenerative disease shown to be proteolytically cleaved by caspase (Goldberg et al., 1996). Htt is predicted to have five sites for caspase cleavage: D513, D552, D586, D530, D859 (Wellington et al., 1998; Wellington et al., 2000). There is no evidence for preferential cleavage of either normal or polyQ-htt, but caspase-mediated cleavage of polyQ-htt has been proposed to generate toxic amino-terminal fragments that may be more toxic than the full length protein, a phenomenon known as toxic fragment hypothesis (Wellington and Hayden, 2000). In addition to caspases, calpains were also found to cleave htt at amino-acids 469 and 536 (Gafni and Ellerby, 2002). Htt is also susceptible to aspartyl proteases that cleave the protein within the amino-terminal domain (Lunkes et al., 2002). A recent study describes the involvement of matrix metalloproteases (MMPs) in the proteolysis of htt at amino-acid 402 (Miller et al., 2010). Finally, Landles and colleagues designed a detailed proteolytic cleavage site map using different antibodies spanning the whole protein and lysates from different brain regions of HD mice (Landles et al., 2010). Proteolytic cleavage of htt is one proposed pathogenic mechanism in HD (see below).

Htt Function

Despite several *in vitro* and *in vivo* studies aimed at elucidating htt function during the last 20 years, the cellular role of htt remains elusive. Htt is a ubiquitous protein expressed at highest levels in the brain and testes (Li et al., 1993; Strong et al., 1993). At the subcellular level, htt predominantly localizes to the cytosol, but it has also been detected in several other compartments, including the nucleus, endoplasmic reticulum, Golgi apparatus, and endosomes (DiFiglia et al., 1995; Gutekunst et al., 1995; Hoffner et al., 2002). Htt has also been observed in axonal processes and at synapses, in association with microtubules, clathrin-coated vesicles, caveolae, and synaptosomes (DiFiglia et al., 1995; Velier et al., 1998). Deletion of htt during development results in embryonic lethality, indicating that htt is essential throughout development (Duyao et al., 1995; Nasir et al., 1995; Zeitlin et al., 1995). On the other hand, its deletion during adulthood in the forebrain and testes results in neuronal degeneration and sterility, highlighting a critical role of the protein in the maintenance and function of these tissues in the adulthood (Dragatsis et al., 2000). Htt has been shown to play a role in several cellular processes.

Normal htt has an anti-apoptotic role – *In vitro* and *in vivo* studies demonstrate that wild type htt plays an anti-apoptotic and neuroprotective role. Overexpression of normal htt in striatum-derived cells protects from apoptosis (Rigamonti et al., 2000; Rigamonti et al., 2001). Primary striatal neurons from transgenic mice overexpressing full length wild type human htt were more protected from excitotoxic stimuli than cultured striatal neurons from non-trangenic litteramates (Leavitt et al., 2006). Specific inactivation of the mouse homologue hungtintin (Hdh) gene by Cre/*loxP* site-specific recombination strategy in the adult forebrain resulted in neurological abnormalities and progressive neurodegeneration, with signs of apoptotic cells in the hippocampus, cortex, and striatum, and lack of axons (Dragatsis et al., 2000). Recently, a pro-survival role of htt has been investigated in non-mammalian HD models. Htt morpholino-injected Zebrafish showed increased cell death, especially in the mid-brain/hind-brain regions of the developing embryos (Diekmann et al., 2009). Investigations of the molecular mechanisms underlying the neuroprotective role of normal htt revealed that htt prevents the activation of caspase-3 and caspase-9 (Rigamonti et al., 2000; Rigamonti et al., 2001). Moreover, htt also reduced the activity of HIP1, a proapoptotic protein able to activate procaspase 8 by sequestering it into a complex together with HIP1 protein interactor (HIPPI) (Gervais et al., 2002). Recently, a novel anti-apoptotic function of htt has been shown by Luo and colleagues (Luo and Rubinsztein, 2009). They demonstrated that htt exerts anti-apoptotic effects by binding to Pak2 and reducing the ability of caspase 3 and caspase 8 to cleave Pak2 and convert it into a mediator of cell death.

Regulation of neuronal gene expression –The interaction of htt with transcription factors suggests that htt is involved in the regulation of gene transcription. In addition to an indirect role in the regulation of gene expression, several evidence demonstrated that htt localizes to the nucleus and binds to DNA to directly repress gene transcription (Benn et al., 2008; Kegel et al., 2002; Zhai et al., 2005). The most well-established example of htt functioning as a transcriptional regulator is its role in the expression of brain-derived neurotrophic factor (BDNF). BDNF is a neurotrophin that supports the survival of existing neurons and promotes the growth and differentiation of new neurons and synapses. In 2001, Zuccato and colleagues observed that wild type htt, but not the mutant protein, increases the levels of BDNF (Zuccato et al., 2001). Moreover, YAC mice overexpressing full length htt showed high levels of BDNF in the cerebral cortex. Normal htt specifically regulates the activity of a BDNF promoter (Zuccato et al., 2007; Zuccato et al., 2003). BDNF promoter contains a silencing DNA response element, the neuron-restrictive silencer element (NRSE, also known as RE1). The RE1/NRSE element is recognized by RE1-silencing transcription factor (REST), also known as neuron-restrictive silencer factor (NRSF). Normal htt indirectly sequesters REST/NRSF into the cytoplasm, thereby preventing the formation of the repressor complex into the nucleus (Zuccato et al., 2007; Zuccato et al., 2003). The effect of normal htt on REST/NRSF-regulated gene expression is not limited to BDNF, as *in vitro* and *in vivo* overexpression of normal htt leads to increased mRNA transcription of several RE1/NRSE-controlled neuronal genes (Zuccato et al., 2007; Zuccato et al., 2003).

Regulation of vesicle and axonal transport – Interactions of htt with several endocytic/trafficking proteins and its localization to endocytic/endosomal vesicles in axons suggest that htt might also be involved in the regulation of intracellular trafficking and endocytosis (Harjes and Wanker, 2003; Li and Li, 2004; Truant et al., 2006). Consistent with this idea, htt binds cytoplasmatic proteins such as huntingtin-associated protein 1 (HAP1) and HIP1, which are involved in microtubule-dependent transport and endocytosis (Engelender et al., 1997; Li et al., 1998; Li et al., 2002b). Data from invertebrate and mammalian models of HD also demonstrate that htt is essential for fast axonal trafficking. Reduction of htt expression in Drosophila has been shown to disrupt axonal transport (Gunawardena et al., 2003). Mice expressing less than 50% htt display severe trafficking defects, suggesting that normal trafficking requires htt (Trushina et al., 2004). Moreover, in 2004 Gauthier and colleagues showed that wild type htt specifically enhances the vesicular transport of BDNF along microtubules in mammalian cells (Gauthier et al., 2004). This idea is further supported by the observation that endogenous wild type htt and BDNF co-localize in neuronal cells (Fusco et al., 2003), and that the transport of BDNF-containing vesicles is increased by overexpression of wild type htt, and, conversely, it is reduced by decreased expression of the protein (Gauthier et al., 2004). The underlying mechanism involves interaction of htt with HAP1, which binds to proteins involved in vesicle transport, such as the p150Glued subunit of dynactin (Gauthier et al., 2004).

Regulation of synaptic transmission - Normal htt is highly expressed at the pre-synaptic level and interacts with cytoskeletal and synaptic vesicle proteins. At the post-synaptic level, normal htt is associated with postsynaptic density protein 95 (PSD-95), a scaffold protein that regulates the clustering and activation of receptors in the postsynaptic membrane (Sun et al., 2001). Overexpression of normal htt has been shown to prevent neuronal toxicity mediated by glutamate receptors by sequestering PSD-95 (Sun et al., 2001). Yeast two hybrid study revealed that SH3-domain GRB2-like 3 (SH3GL3) selectively interacts with htt in a polyQ length-dependent manner (Sittler et al., 1998). In the central nervous system, SH3-containing proteins play a major role in the signal transduction from membrane receptors and in the regulation of the exo/endocytic cycle of synaptic vesicles. Htt also directly binds to protein kinase C and casein kinase 2 substrate in neurons (PACSIN 1), which plays a central role in synaptic vesicle recycling (Modregger et al., 2002).

Molecular Mechanisms of HD Pathogenesis

HD has been proposed to either result from a dominant-negative effect of mutant htt on the wild type counterpart, which leads to a loss of protein function, or from a novel, toxic gain of function of mutant protein. Expansion of the polyQ tract in htt alters several cellular processes, ultimately leading to neuronal cell dysfunction and death.

Misfolding and Aggregation of polyQ-htt - The formation of neuronal intranuclear and intracytoplasmtic inclusions of polyQ-htt is a pathological hallmark of HD. The first evidence of abnormal nuclear structures in brain specimens from HD patients dates back to the seventies (Roizin et al., 1974). Subsequently, intranuclear inclusions were found in transgenic mice expressing the first exon of the human HD gene (Davies et al., 1997). Immunostaining with an antibody that detects expanded polyQ tracts revealed the presence of circular, densely stained intraneuronal inclusions. These nuclear inclusions observed in the striatum, cerebral cortex, cerebellum and spinal cord also showed ubiquitin-positive reactivity. More recently, intranuclear inclusions have been described in a large set of HD transgenic mice over expressing full-length or truncated forms of the expanded protein as well as in many other animal models including *Drosophila Melanogaster* and *C. Elegans*. In 1997, Di Figlia and colleagues confirmed the presence and features of the intranuclear ubiquitin-positive inclusions in human HD brain (DiFiglia, 1997). Although all these initial reports described inclusions primarily in the nucleus of HD brain neurons, further studies also reported their presence in the cytoplasm and in neuronal processes (Cooper et al., 1998; Hackam et al., 1998; Martindale et al., 1998). Moreover, the formation, localization and frequency of these inclusions are influenced by the htt fragment length and amount (Cooper et al., 1998; Hackam et al., 1998;

Martindale et al., 1998), as well as by the polyQ tract length (Hackam et al., 1998; Li and Li, 1998; Martindale et al., 1998).

The central role of aggregation and inclusion formation as toxic pathogenetic events in HD and other neurodegenerative disorders has recently been questioned by several studies, and the question as to whether polyQ-htt aggregates and inclusions are deleterious, harmless or protective remains unsolved. The toxicity of aggregates and inclusions is based on the evidence that there is a strong correlation between aggregate formation and cell death in mammalian cell culture systems (Hackam et al., 1998; Ho et al., 2001). Consistent with the *in vitro* data, aggregation increases with disease progression also in HD mouse models (Yamamoto et al., 2000). It has been proposed that toxicity results from the sequestration into aggregates and inclusions of several cellular proteins, such as transcription factors and transcriptional regulators (Nucifora et al., 2001; Steffan et al., 2000), ubiquitin-proteasome system components (Davies et al., 1997; Jana et al., 2000; Waelter et al., 2001; Wyttenbach et al., 2000), and soluble motor proteins (Gunawardena et al., 2003; Li et al., 2001; Parker et al., 2001). Therefore, recruitment of proteins into inclusions might trigger different pathogenetic processes, including not only transcriptional dysregulation and proteasome impairment, but also axonal transport and synaptic transmission because of their abilities to sequester soluble motor proteins. On the other hand, several studies reported dissociation between aggregation/inclusion formation and toxicity, supporting the idea that inclusions are not pathogenic. Rather, inclusions may represent an attempt of the cells to sequester toxic soluble fragments (Kuemmerle et al., 1999). One of the most striking evidence in support of this idea comes from a longitudinal survival analysis of HD primary striatal neurons, in which those cells forming large htt inclusions had an increased survival rate compared to those not forming any inclusions (Arrasate et al., 2004). Also in HD mouse models, the presence of inclusions containing polyQ-htt and toxicity are events that may be independent from each other (Slow et al., 2005).

A new hypothesis to reconcile both toxic and protective roles of inclusions/aggregation has been proposed. Micro-aggregates, oligomeric forms or even aberrantly misfolded monomeric forms of polyQ-htt have been proposed to be toxic species, while large inclusions sequestering these diffuse toxic forms have been proposed to be protective species (Arrasate et al., 2004; Beal et al., 1991; Bennett et al., 2007).

Defects in polyQ-htt clearance - Cells have evolved two mechanisms for the degradation of misfolded proteins: the ubiquitin–proteasome system (UPS) and lysosome-mediated autophagy.

UPS involves a three step process, whereby a target protein is covalently conjugated to a poly-ubiquitin chain, recognized by the proteasome and degraded within its core. The observation that polyQ-htt inclusions colocalize with ubiquitin and proteasome components in HD cell and mouse models and in HD patient-derived specimens (Davies et al., 1997; DiFiglia, 1997; Jana et al., 2000; Waelter et al., 2001; Wyttenbach et al., 2000) suggested that polyQ-htt is targeted for degradation, but it cannot be properly cleared because the UPS is dysfunctional. The impairment of the UPS in HD has been observed in different cellular models (Bence et al., 2001; Jana et al., 2001; Maynard et al., 2009), in HD mouse models (Bennett et al., 2007; Wang et al., 2008), and in human tissues (Bennett et al., 2007; Seo et al., 2004). The decreased UPS activity in HD has been proposed to be due to the sequestration of UPS components into aggregates, thereby resulting in altered subcellular localization (Jana et al., 2001). Alternatively, proteins containing an expanded polyQ tract could not be cleaved properly by the proteasome, and the uncleaved polyQ tract trapped into the proteasome might block the entry of other substrates into the barrel of the proteasome catalytic core (Holmberg et al., 2004; Venkatraman et al., 2004). However, several studies reported that the UPS is not impaired in HD (Bowman et al., 2005; Ding et al., 2002), and other studies rather demonstrated an increase in proteasome activity (Bett et al., 2006; Diaz-Hernandez et al., 2003; Seo et al., 2008).

Autophagy involves cell degradation of unwanted or dysfunctional cellular components through the lysosomal machinery. During this process, targeted cytoplasmic constituents are entrapped into double-membrane structures called autophagosomes, which then fuse with lysosomes and are degraded or recycled. Autophagy plays a critical role in the clearance of polyQ-htt (Kegel et al., 2000; Petersen et al., 2001; Qin et al., 2003; Ravikumar et al., 2002). Ravikumar and colleagues reported that the negative regulator of the autophagic pathway, mechanistic target of rapamycin (mTOR), colocalizes with aggregated polyQ-htt in HD cellular models, transgenic mice, and patient-derived brain specimens (Ravikumar et al., 2004). More recently, Heng and co-workers demonstrated that the expression levels of two autophagy proteins, the ubiquitin-binding protein p62 (p62) and the light chain 3-II (LC3-II) are increased at early stages of disease in a new HD mouse model (Su et al., 2010). Moreover, the lysosome-associated membrane protein type 2A (LAMP-2A) and lysosomal heat shock protein 70 (hsc70) are markedly increased in HD models (Koga et al., 2011). Pharmacological inhibition of autophagy in HD cell models enhanced htt aggregation and toxicity (Ravikumar et al., 2002). Consistent with these observations, stimulation of autophagy or overexpression of factors involved in autophagy reduced aggregation, increased the clearance of polyQ-htt and improved the phenotype of mouse, Drosophila, and C. Elegans HD models (Bauer et al., 2010; Ho et al., 2001; Ravikumar et al., 2004; Rose et al., 2010; Tsvetkov et al., 2010). Trafficking of polyQ-htt into autophagosomes can be promoted by acetylation of polyQ-htt at lysine residue 444 (K444), suggesting that acetylation of htt is necessary for its degradation via autophagy, and this post-translational modification is increased in polyQ-htt (Jeong et al., 2009). More recently, Martinez-Vincente and colleagues identified a primary defect in the ability of autophagic vacuoles to recognize cytosolic cargo in HD cells (Martinez-Vicente et al., 2010).

Proteolytic Cleavage - Several evidence supports the idea that a key step in HD pathogenesis is the aberrant polyQ-htt cleavage that generates toxic fragments containing expanded polyQ tracts (Wellington and Hayden, 2000). Htt-truncated fragments have been detected in cell models of HD (Ratovitski et al., 2007), in mouse models expressing full length polyQ-htt (Gray et al., 2008; Hodgson et al., 1999; Tanaka et al., 2006), and in HD postmortem tissues (Lunkes et al., 2002). Notably, mouse models generated with an amino-terminal htt fragment showed a more severe phenotype than mice expressing full-length htt (Waldron-Roby et al., 2012). Elevated caspase activity has been observed in neuronal cell lines expressing polyQ-htt as well as in brain samples from HD mouse models and HD patients, and treatment with caspase inhibitors reduced polyQ-htt toxicity (Gafni et al., 2004; Graham et al., 2010; Hermel et al., 2004; Kim et al., 1999). To determine if caspase cleavage or the resulting fragments are critical for HD pathogenesis, Graham and colleagues generated transgenic mice expressing caspase-3- and caspase-6-resistant polyQ-htt (Graham et al., 2006). They showed that mice expressing a polyQ-htt variant resistant to cleavage by caspase-6, but not caspase-3, maintain normal neuronal function and do not develop striatal neurodegeneration. Gafni and coworkers reported an elevated calpain activity in HD mouse brains and HD patients that could result from increased calcium influx into neurons after excitotoxic stimuli (Gafni and Ellerby, 2002; Gafni et al., 2004). Moreover, inhibition of calpain cleavage reduced toxicity in HD cells (Gafni and Ellerby, 2002; Gafni et al., 2004). Elevated matrix metalloproteinase (MMP) levels were found in HD mouse models and prevention of metallo-proteinase cleavage by knocking down MMP-10 rescued striatal neurons expressing polyQ-htt from cell death (Miller et al., 2010).

Mitochondrial Dysfunction – Metabolic defects, such as weight loss, early alterations of brain homeostasis, and altered cerebral glucose uptake and consumption, have been reported in HD patients (Antonini et al., 1996; Jenkins et al., 1993; Kuhl et al., 1982; Leenders et al., 1986) and HD mouse models (Browne et al., 1999; Mangiarini et al., 1996), thereby linking HD pathogenesis to mitochondrial dysfunction. PolyQ-htt has been reported to affect mitochondrial function by multiple mechanisms, including reduction of energy production and membrane potential, alteration of calcium homeostasis, enhancement of oxidative stress and impairment of transcription of genes involved in the functioning and biogenesis of this organelle. Several biochemical studies on the brain of HD patients, cells, and animal models revealed an impaired activity of respiratory chain complexes and tricarboxilic acid (TCA) cycle enzymes (Browne, 2008). Mitochondria are the major source of reactive oxygen species (ROS) and, at the same time, they are also a key target for ROS damage. To protect cells against damage caused by ROS, mitochondria contain several antioxidant systems and enzymatic components. PolyQ-htt expression has been linked to excessive production of ROS or disruption of the antioxidant mechanisms, leading to oxidative damage of mitochondrial proteins, lipids, and DNA (Hands et al., 2011; Li et al., 2010; Wyttenbach et al., 2002). On the other hand, oxidative damage can cause somatic expansions of the CAG repeat tract in post-mitotic neurons, resulting in a longer and more toxic polyQ expanded htt (Kovtun et al., 2007). Several studies on mitochondria from HD patient lymphoblasts, HD mouse brain and neuronal cell lines support a role for mitochondrial calcium handling defects in HD pathogenesis (Choo et al., 2004; Chopra et al., 2007; Oliveira et al., 2006; Panov et al., 2003; Panov et al., 2002).

Another HD-specific mechanism that could mediate mitochondrial dysfunction is the reduction of expression of peroxisome proliferator-activated receptor-γ co-activator 1α (PGC-1α) (Cui et al., 2006). PGC-1α is a transcriptional coactivator that regulates several metabolic processes, including mitochondrial biogenesis and oxidative function. In HD, PGC-1α levels and activity are impaired in the brain and muscles of patients and transgenic mice (Chaturvedi et al., 2009; Cui et al., 2006; Weydt et al., 2006). Polymorphisms in PPARGC1A, the gene encoding PGC-1α, have been associated with altered age of onset of HD, further implying a role for mitochondrial defects in HD (Che et al., 2011; Weydt et al., 2009). Recently, several studies demonstrated that expression of PGC-1α partially reverses the toxic effects of polyQ-htt in cultured striatal neurons (Cui et al., 2006; Weydt et al., 2006).

Transcriptional Dysregulation – The idea that transcription dysregulation is critical in HD pathogenesis came from analysis of gene expression in HD human post mortem brain specimens and in HD mouse models (Cha, 2007). Early in situ hybridization studies on post mortem human brains revealed that specific mRNA products encoding signaling neuropeptides and neurotransmitter receptors were decreased in HD specimens (Arzberger et al., 1997; Augood et al., 1997; Augood et al., 1996; Norris et al., 1996). Glutamate receptor levels in R6/2 mice have been shown to be decreased, as were dopamine D1 and D2 receptors in brain (Cha et al., 1999; Cha et al., 1998). Subsequently, several other single-gene studies performed in several HD mouse models confirmed transcriptional alterations in HD. Most of these gene expression alterations were detected in transgenic mice expressing only exon 1 of human htt, suggesting that such transcriptional changes may be related to the expansion of the polyQ tract and, as such, may be common to other polyQ diseases (Ross, 2002). A more comprehensive analysis of gene expression changes in HD transgenic mouse models was performed using the microarray technology. In 2000, the Hereditary Disease Array Group (HDAG) generated a gene expression HD database, which led to the identification of groups of genes involved in transcriptional processes, neurotransmitter receptors, synaptic transmission, cytoskeletal and structural proteins, intracellular signaling and calcium homeostasis, whose expression is altered in HD (Chan et al., 2002; Fossale et al., 2002; Luthi-Carter et al., 2002a; Luthi-Carter et al., 2002b; Sipione et al., 2002). Gene expression analysis was also carried out in several HD cell models and brought to the identification of novel gene pathways altered in HD, such as cholesterol biogenesis (Apostol et al., 2006; Kita et al., 2002; Sipione et al., 2002; Sugars et al., 2004; Valenza et al., 2005; Wyttenbach et al., 2001).

Several mechanisms have been proposed to explain how polyQ-htt alters gene expression. PolyQ-htt may directly affect the activity of transcription factors, as several transcription factors were shown to bind htt in a polyQ length-dependent manner (Dunah et al., 2002; Li et al., 2002a; Nucifora et al., 2001; Steffan et al., 2000; Zuccato et al., 2007; Zuccato et al., 2003). Moreover, Zhai and coworkers identified the two components of the transcriptional machinery, transcription factor II D (TFIID) and transcription factor II F (TFIIF), as direct targets of polyQ-htt, suggesting that polyQ expansions in htt disrupts the function of the core transcriptional machinery (Zhai et al., 2005). However, transcriptional machinery factors such as the

RNA polymerase II large subunit can be also be sequestered into inclusions formed by expanded polyQ proteins (Luthi-Carter et al., 2002b). PolyQ-htt also directly binds the acetyltransferase domain of CBP and p300/CBP associated factor (P/CAF), blocking their acetyltransferase activity and leading to a condensed chromatin state and reduced gene expression (Steffan et al., 2001). Finally, recent studies have shown that the microRNA system is altered in HD (Gaughwin et al., 2011; Ghose et al., 2011; Jin et al., 2012; Johnson et al., 2008; Packer et al., 2008).

Transport defects –Two independent studies performed on invertebrate models demonstrated impaired axonal transport in transgenic Drosophila models of HD (Gunawardena et al., 2003; Lee et al., 2004). In addition, expression of full-length polyQ-htt impaired vesicular and mitochondrial trafficking in mammalian neurons *in vitro* and *in vivo* (Trushina et al., 2004). BDNF vesicular transport in neuronal cells has been shown to be attenuated in HD (Gauthier et al., 2004; Her and Goldstein, 2008). Constitutive phosphorylation of polyQ-htt at serine 421 (S421) restored its function in axonal transport by promoting the interaction between htt and the p150(Glued) subunit of dynactin and their association with microtubules (Zala et al., 2008). How does polyQ-htt interfere with cellular transport? Expansion of polyQ in htt alters the interaction of htt with several proteins involved in vesicular trafficking (Kalchman et al., 1997; Li et al., 1995; Modregger et al., 2002; Peters and Ross, 2001; Singaraja et al., 2002), as well as it alters the expression of proteins that regulate vesicle transport (Hodges et al., 2006; Sipione et al., 2002). In addition, polyQ-htt aggregation can block axonal transport due to the accumulation of material along the axons (Chang et al., 2006; Lee et al., 2004), or it can sequester proteins required for vesicle transport (Caviston and Holzbaur, 2009).

Excitotoxicity - Excitotoxicity is a pathological process that leads to neuronal death upon excessive stimulation by neurotransmitters, such as glutamate. In the context of HD, neuronal dysfunction and death of striatal medium-sized spiny neurons have been shown to result from excessive activation of glutamate receptors due to increased glutamate release from cortical afferents and reduced uptake of glutamate by glia (Fan and Raymond, 2007). The idea that excitotoxicity plays a role in HD pathogenesis came from large evidence of glutamatergic neurotransmission dysfunction in autoptic HD human brain. Neurons expressing glutamate receptors in human HD striatum are lost early in disease (Albin et al., 1990; London et al., 1981; Young et al., 1988). In addition, striatal injection of agonists selective for *N*-methyl-d-aspartate (NMDA)-type glutamate receptors in rats and non-human primates reproduced the neurochemical and neuropathological changes seen in HD (Beal et al., 1986; Sanberg et al., 1989; Schwarcz et al., 1984). Consistent with the excitotoxic hypothesis, examination of the electrophysiological responsiveness of NMDA receptors at the cellular level in two different HD transgenic models demonstrated altered NMDA receptor function in HD (Cepeda et al., 2001; Levine et al., 1999). Moreover, Zeron and colleagues found that striatal medium-sized spiny neurons from YAC46 and YAC72 mice showed increased vulnerability to NMDA-induced apoptosis from birth in comparison to wild type controls (Zeron et al., 2004; Zeron et al., 2002). However, R6/1 and R6/2 HD mice have been shown to be more resistant to excitotoxic insults than wild type mice (Hansson et al., 1999; Morton and Leavens, 2000). Transgenic mice that develop resistance against excitotoxicity were those that showed an accelerated HD phenotype and expressed only a truncated version of htt, comprising the N-terminal portion including the polyQ tract. Changes in NMDA receptors (NMDAR) protein levels in autoptic HD human brain and in HD mouse models have been proposed as a mechanism underlying altered NMDAR activity in HD (Ali and Levine, 2006; Benn et al., 2007; Cepeda et al., 2001; Cha et al., 1999; Jarabek et al., 2004).

Clinical Perspectives in HD

All the HD pathogenic pathways that have been emerging in the last years offer therapeutic targets for potential treatments. In 2008, the U.S. Food and Drug Administration approved tetrabenazine as the first drug to treat HD patients. However, all the strategies pursued so far to treat HD patients, including tetrabenazine, may help to alleviate symptoms, but there is no currently treatment available to stop or reverse the course of disease (Armstrong et al., 2012). Here, we will discuss the HD therapeutic strategies currently under development focusing on their specific targets.

Targeting aggregation – Preventing the formation of polyQ-htt aggregation in neurons represents an attractive therapeutic strategy to ameliorate HD. The first high-throughput screening for small molecules suppressing polyQ-htt into aggregation has been developed in 2002 by Heiser and colleagues (Heiser et al., 2002). Using an automated filter retardation assay for the rapid identification of chemical compounds that prevent HD exon 1 aggregation *in vitro*, they found that riluzole significantly inhibits polyQ-htt aggregation in a dose-dependent manner. Despite the contrasting results obtained upon treatment of HD mice (Hockly et al., 2006; Schiefer et al., 2002), riluzole has been tested in clinical trial (Landwehrmeyer et al., 2007). Later, a yeast-based high-throughput screening assay has been applied to identify aggregation inhibitors in HD (Zhang et al., 2005). The isolated compound, an epigallocatechin-3-gallate, C2-8, inhibited polyQ aggregation in cell cultures and brain slices, rescued degeneration of photoreceptors in a Drosophila model of HD, and improved motor performance by reducing neuronal atrophy and polyQ-htt aggregation in HD mice (Chopra et al., 2007). Recently, a luciferase-based protein aggregation reporter assay identified leflunomide and teriflunomide as polyQ aggregation inhibitors (Fuentealba et al., 2012). The azo-dye Congo red, a known inhibitor of oligomerization, prevented ATP depletion and caspase activation, preserved normal cellular protein synthesis and degradation functions, and promoted the clearance of expanded polyQ repeats *in vitro* and *in vivo* (Sanchez et al., 2003). Recently, methilene blue has been shown to modulate polyQ-htt aggregation intermediates and protect from the toxicity of mutant protein (Sontag et al., 2012).

Clearance of Htt – Accelerating the degradation of polyQ-htt might be a potential therapeutic strategy for HD. Several studies have shown that enhancement of proteasome degradation by overexpression/activation of heat shock proteins or chaperones reduces polyQ-htt aggregation and increases the survival in HD Drosophila and mouse models (Carmichael et al., 2000; Vacher et al., 2005; Warrick et al., 1999; Wyttenbach et al., 2000). A high-throughput screen aimed at identifying molecules that enhance degradation or clearance of soluble polyQ-htt has led to the discovery of a class of compounds that facilitate the clearance of polyQ-htt by the UPS (Baldo et al., 2012).

Activation of autophagy may also offer protection in HD by increasing the clearance of polyQ-htt-positive inclusions (Sarkar and Rubinsztein, 2008). Pharmacological inhibition of autophagy in HD cell models enhanced polyQ-htt aggregation formation and toxicity (Ravikumar et al., 2002). Consistent with this observation, stimulation of autophagy or overexpression of factors involved in autophagy reduced aggregation, increased the clearance of polyQ-htt in HD cellular models, and improved the phenotype of mouse, fly, and C. Elegans models (Ho et al., 2001; Ravikumar et al., 2004; Rose et al., 2010; Sarkar et al., 2007; Tsvetkov et al., 2010; Williams et al., 2008). Autophagy is negatively regulated by mTOR. In particular, inhibition of mTOR by rapamycin resulted in autophagy activation and reduced toxicity of polyQ-htt in fly and mouse models of HD (Ravikumar et al., 2004). Autophagy can also be induced by lowering intracellular inositol or IP3 levels independently of mTOR. Lithium induces autophagy by reducing intracellular inositol levels, and this has been shown to reduce polyQ-htt aggregation/toxicity in HD cell models and protect against neurodegeneration in HD Drosophila models (Sarkar et al., 2005; Sarkar et al., 2008). An *in vitro* screening to search for compounds able to inhibit polyQ-mediated protein aggregation identified the disaccharide trehalose (Tanaka et al., 2004). Trehalose has been found to reduce aggregation and toxicity of polyQ-htt in HD cells, to protect from pro-apoptotic insults and to attenuate disease manifestations in HD mice by enhancing autophagy pathways independently of mTOR (Sarkar et al., 2007; Tanaka et al., 2004).

Targeting mitochondrial dysfunction – PolyQ expansions in htt are associated with mitochondrial dysfunction, resulting in impaired energy production, increased intracellular calcium, oxidative stress and apoptosis. However, several drugs that increase mitochondrial function, such as creatine, coenzyme Q and the omega-3-derived fatty acid, ethyl-eicosapentaenoic acid (ethyl-EPA), have been tested in clinical trials without much success. The limited success of these studies could be due to the poor pharmacokinetic properties of the tested compounds and to the underestimation of the optimal therapeutic dose (Handley et al., 2006). Although creatine and coenzyme Q, which stimulate mitochondrial respiration and have antioxidant properties, both alleviated pathologic symptoms in HD mouse models (Andreassen et al., 2001; Ferrante et al., 2002; Ferrante et al., 2000; Schilling et al., 2001), they did not show any significant benefit in HD patients (Hersch et al., 2006; Huntington Study, 2001; Tabrizi et al., 2005). Treatment of an HD mouse model with ethyl-EPA improved motor function and increased survival (Clifford et al., 2002; Van Raamsdonk et al., 2005). The beneficial effects of EPA on motor function may result from EPA's anti-inflammatory activity or ability to improve mitochondrial function. Several clinical trials have been carried out to test the protective role of EPA in HD, but the efficacy of ethyl-EPA treatment in HD remains unclear (Huntington Study Group, 2008; Puri et al., 2002; Puri et al., 2005).

Restoring gene transcription and BDNF levels – Several compounds have been proposed to ameliorate HD phenotype in animal models by restoring normal transcription levels. Histone deacetylase (HDAC) inhibitors increase histone acetylation leading to a less compact and transcriptionally more active chromatin and have been investigated with therapeutic purposes in HD flies (Steffan et al., 2001). HDAC inhibitors, such as suberoylanilide hydroxamatic acid (SAHA), sodium butyrate and phenylbutirate, may represent a means to attenuate HD phenotype by improving transcriptional regulation. Several preclinical studies in HD mouse models have been carried out using different HDAC inhibitors, confirming the neuroprotective effect observed in invertebrates (Ferrante et al., 2003; Gardian et al., 2005; Hockly et al., 2003; Thomas et al., 2008). Notably, the neuroprotective effects of HDAC inhibitors have also been attributed to the anti-aggregation, anti-inflammatory and anti-apoptotic properties of these compounds (Goffredo et al., 2002; Iwata et al., 2005). Although a clinical trial on HD patients revealed that sodium phenylbutyrate is safe and well tolerated in humans (Hogarth et al., 2007), HDAC inhibitors are highly toxic and further studies are needed to clarify their biological functions and their specific targets.

The observation that reduced levels of BDNF contribute to HD pathogenesis suggested that BDNF administration is a potential therapeutic approach for HD (Zuccato et al., 2001). In the last decade, several experimental strategies have been applied with the attempt to restore the BDNF levels in HD, including BDNF infusion, gene therapy, BDNF releasing cell grafts, BDNF mimetics, specific diet and drugs (Zuccato and Cattaneo, 2009). Although the promising results obtained in preclinical studies on HD animal models, many issues regarding the dosage and the delivery method of BDNF therapy remain to be investigated.

Targeting excitotoxicity –The only approved drug for HD is tetrabenazine, a vescicular monoamine transporter-2 (VMAT2) inhibitor that lowers extracellular dopamine and norepinephrine (Frank et al., 2008; Huntington Study, 2006). However, despite its beneficial effect on chorea, tetrabenazine has many side effects and fails to improve the cognitive and psychiatric deficits or to slow HD progression. This compound alleviates motor deficits and reduces striatal cell death in HD mice, confirming that the dopamine signaling pathway plays an important role in HD pathogenesis (Tang et al., 2007; Wang et al., 2010).

A different approach to counteract excitotoxicity in HD brain is to block the excessive glutamate released from cortico-striatal terminals. Murine HD models showed increased survival upon treatment with the NMDA receptor antagonist riluzole (Schiefer et al., 2002). However, three different human clinical trials conducted in HD patients treated with riluzole reported opposing results (Landwehrmeyer et al., 2007; Rosas et al., 1999; Seppi et al., 2001). The most recent one, a 3 years randomized controlled study carried out in almost 400 Europeans HD patients, showed no neuroprotective or beneficial effects of riluzole in HD (Landwehrmeyer et al., 2007). Memantine, another NMDA receptor antagonist, was tested in HD patients and the results suggested that memantine treatment of HD may be useful to delay disease progression (Beister et al., 2004; Ondo et al., 2007).

Lamotrigine, a glutamate antagonist, and remacemide, a non-competitive inhibitor of the NMDA receptors, have also been tested in human clinical trials, but they were associated with many side effects and no significant improvement of disease phenotype was observed (Huntington Study, 2001; Kieburtz et al., 1996; Kremer et al., 1999).

Targeting mutant Htt – The strategies described above to counteract HD are indirect and function downstream the effects of polyQ-htt. Moreover, all these approaches are aimed to target specifically just one or few pathogenic functions of polyQ-htt. An interesting strategy for treating HD is based on the possibility to block the production of polyQ-htt by targeting either the mRNA or the protein. Oligonucleotides such as RNAi and antisense oligonucleotides (ASOs) directly targeting polyQ-htt mRNA could be feasible strategies in the treatment of HD (Sah and Aronin, 2011). Partial lowering of polyQ-htt through ASOs and duplex RNAs (dsRNAs) has been shown to alleviate symptoms and prolong survival in HD models (Boudreau et al., 2009; DiFiglia et al., 2007; Drouet et al., 2009; Harper et al., 2005). Although normal htt plays significant roles in the adult brain, these studies indicated that reduction of htt can be tolerated in mice up to 9 months. Moreover, reduction of both normal and polyQ-htt by ASOs in HD mice had the same benefits as reduction of polyQ-htt alone (Kordasiewicz et al., 2012). Accordingly, partial suppression of wild type htt in the brain of non-human primates has been reported to be safe (McBride et al., 2011). However, further investigations addressing a long term-neuronal tolerance for reduction of normal htt are necessary. Strategies to selectively silence the polyQ-htt-encoding allele have been applied. Allele-specific silencing of polyQ-htt is achieved by targeting associated single nucleotide polymorphisms (SNPs) (Lombardi et al., 2009; Pfister et al., 2009; van Bilsen et al., 2008; Warby et al., 2009). An alternative approach for allele-selective inhibition strategy takes advantages of a universal difference between the mutant and the wild type alleles, which is the polyQ repeat length. Recently, Yu and colleagues described potent and allele-selective inhibition of polyQ-htt expression in HD patient-derived cells and HD mice using single-strand siRNAs (ss-siRNAs) targeting the CAG repeat (Yu et al., 2012).

Intracellular antibodies (intrabodies) provide a protein-based approach to targeting polyQ-htt (Butler et al., 2012). Intrabodies are small, recombinant antibody fragments that target antigens intracellularly via the Fv variable regions that are responsible for antibody specificity. Based on the fact that expression of polyQ-htt exon1 is sufficient to cause HD in several animal models, intrabodies directed towards the three domains of htt exon1 (the N-17 AA, the polyQ tract and the proline-rich region) have been created. The initial target of intrabody-based therapy was the polyQ repeat, but these antibodies increased toxicity likely by stabilizing a toxic conformation (Khoshnan et al., 2002). The first intrabody that successfully counteracted polyQ-htt aggregation and toxicity *in vitro* was scFv-C4, which is specific for the 17 N-terminal residues of htt (Lecerf et al., 2001; Murphy and Messer, 2004). This intrabody has also been tested in HD Drosophila and mouse models, where it has been shown to reduce aggregation and extend life span in HD flies (Snyder-Keller et al., 2010; Wolfgang et al., 2005). A series of intrabodies against the proline-rich region of htt has also been developed (Ko et al., 2001; Southwell et al., 2008). Adeno-associated virus 2/1 intrastriatal delivery of Happ1 intrabody, specific for the proline-rich domain, ameliorated motor, cognitive and neuropathological symptoms in several HD mouse models (Southwell et al., 2009).

Conclusion

The discovery of polyQ expansion in the gene encoding huntingtin as the mutation responsible for HD dates to the early 1990s (1993). Two decades later, however, there is no effective therapy for HD and the other neurodegenerative diseases caused by expanded polyQ. Although it has been already demonstrated that HD is mainly caused by a toxic gain of function due to polyQ expansion, multiple models suggest that also a loss of function of wild type htt may contribute significantly to several aspects of disease pathogenesis. During the last 20 years, significant achievements in our understanding of the pathogenesis of HD have been reached. However, more efforts are needed to clearly identify the main functions of normal htt and the most critical pathways for neurodegeneration in HD. From a therapeutic point of view, new discoveries improving knowledge of htt biology and identifying novel pathogenic pathways may represent a worthwhile avenue to pursue for development of therapy for HD.

Acknowledgments

This work was supported by Telethon-Italy (GGP10037), the Muscular Dystrophy Association (196646), the Kennedy's Disease Association, and a Marie-Curie Reintegration Grant (FP7-256448).

Conflict of Interest

M.P. received support from Siena Biotech (Italy). The authors have no conflict of interest to declare.

References

<The Hungtington's diesease collaborative research group, 1993.pdf>.

(1993). A novel gene containing a trinucleotide repeat that is expanded and unstable on Huntington's disease chromosomes. The Huntington's Disease Collaborative Research Group. *Cell 72*, 971-983.

Aiken, C.T., Steffan, J.S., Guerrero, C.M., Khashwji, H., Lukacsovich, T., Simmons, D., Purcell, J.M., Menhaji, K., Zhu, Y.Z., Green, K., *et al.* (2009). Phosphorylation of threonine 3: implications for Huntingtin aggregation and neurotoxicity. *J. Biol. Chem. 284*, 29427-29436.

Albin, R.L., Young, A.B., Penney, J.B., Handelin, B., Balfour, R., Anderson, K.D., Markel, D.S., Tourtellotte, W.W., and Reiner, A. (1990). Abnormalities of striatal projection neurons and N-methyl-D-aspartate receptors in presymptomatic Huntington's disease. *The New England journal of medicine 322*, 1293-1298.

Ali, N.J., and Levine, M.S. (2006). Changes in expression of N-methyl-D-aspartate receptor subunits occur early in the R6/2 mouse model of Huntington's disease. *Dev. Neurosci. 28*, 230-238.

Andreassen, O.A., Dedeoglu, A., Ferrante, R.J., Jenkins, B.G., Ferrante, K.L., Thomas, M., Friedlich, A., Browne, S.E., Schilling, G., Borchelt, D.R., *et al.* (2001). Creatine Increases Survival and Delays Motor Symptoms in a Transgenic Animal Model of Huntington's Disease. *Neurobiology of Disease 8*, 479-491.

Anne, S.L., Saudou, F., and Humbert, S. (2007). Phosphorylation of huntingtin by cyclin-dependent kinase 5 is induced by DNA damage and regulates wild-type and mutant huntingtin toxicity in neurons. *J. Neurosci. 27*, 7318-7328.

Antonini, A., Leenders, K.L., Spiegel, R., Meier, D., Vontobel, P., Weigell-Weber, M., Sanchez-Pernaute, R., de Yebenez, J.G., Boesiger, P., Weindl, A., *et al.* (1996). Striatal glucose metabolism and dopamine D2 receptor binding in asymptomatic gene carriers and patients with Huntington's disease. *Brain : a journal of neurology 119 (Pt 6)*, 2085-2095.

Apostol, B.L., Illes, K., Pallos, J., Bodai, L., Wu, J., Strand, A., Schweitzer, E.S., Olson, J.M., Kazantsev, A., Marsh, J.L., *et al.* (2006). Mutant huntingtin alters MAPK signaling pathways in PC12 and striatal cells: ERK1/2 protects against mutant huntingtin-associated toxicity. *Hum. Mol. Genet. 15*, 273-285.

Armstrong, M.J., Miyasaki, J.M., and American Academy of, N. (2012). Evidence-based guideline: pharmacologic treatment of chorea in Huntington disease: report of the guideline development subcommittee of the American Academy of Neurology. *Neurology 79*, 597-603.

Arrasate, M., Mitra, S., Schweitzer, E.S., Segal, M.R., and Finkbeiner, S. (2004). Inclusion body formation reduces levels of mutant huntingtin and the risk of neuronal death. *Nature 431*, 805-810.

Arzberger, T., Krampfl, K., Leimgruber, S., and Weindl, A. (1997). Changes of NMDA receptor subunit (NR1, NR2B) and glutamate transporter (GLT1) mRNA expression in Huntington's disease--an in situ hybridization study. *J. Neuropathol. Exp. Neurol. 56*, 440-454.

Atwal, R.S., Xia, J., Pinchev, D., Taylor, J., Epand, R.M., and Truant, R. (2007). Huntingtin has a membrane association signal that can modulate huntingtin aggregation, nuclear entry and toxicity. *Hum. Mol. Genet. 16*, 2600-2615.

Augood, S.J., Faull, R.L., and Emson, P.C. (1997). Dopamine D1 and D2 receptor gene expression in the striatum in Huntington's disease. *Ann. Neurol. 42*, 215-221.

Augood, S.J., Faull, R.L., Love, D.R., and Emson, P.C. (1996). Reduction in enkephalin and substance P messenger RNA in the striatum of early grade Huntington's disease: a detailed cellular in situ hybridization study. *Neuroscience 72*, 1023-1036.

Baldo, B., Weiss, A., Parker, C.N., Bibel, M., Paganetti, P., and Kaupmann, K. (2012). A screen for enhancers of clearance identifies huntingtin as a heat shock protein 90 (Hsp90) client protein. *J. Biol. Chem. 287*, 1406-1414.

Bauer, P.O., Goswami, A., Wong, H.K., Okuno, M., Kurosawa, M., Yamada, M., Miyazaki, H., Matsumoto, G., Kino, Y., Nagai, Y., *et al.* (2010).

Harnessing chaperone-mediated autophagy for the selective degradation of mutant huntingtin protein. *Nat. Biotechnol. 28*, 256-263.

Beal, M.F., Ferrante, R.J., Swartz, K.J., and Kowall, N.W. (1991). Chronic quinolinic acid lesions in rats closely resemble Huntington's disease. *J. Neurosci. 11*, 1649-1659.

Beal, M.F., Kowall, N.W., Ellison, D.W., Mazurek, M.F., Swartz, K.J., and Martin, J.B. (1986). Replication of the neurochemical characteristics of Huntington's disease by quinolinic acid. *Nature 321*, 168-171.

Beister, A., Kraus, P., Kuhn, W., Dose, M., Weindl, A., and Gerlach, M. (2004). The N-methyl-D-aspartate antagonist memantine retards progression of Huntington's disease. *Journal of neural transmission Supplementum,* 117-122.

Bence, N.F., Sampat, R.M., and Kopito, R.R. (2001). Impairment of the ubiquitin-proteasome system by protein aggregation. *Science 292*, 1552-1555.

Benn, C.L., Slow, E.J., Farrell, L.A., Graham, R., Deng, Y., Hayden, M.R., and Cha, J.H. (2007). Glutamate receptor abnormalities in the YAC128 transgenic mouse model of Huntington's disease. *Neuroscience 147*, 354-372.

Benn, C.L., Sun, T., Sadri-Vakili, G., McFarland, K.N., DiRocco, D.P., Yohrling, G.J., Clark, T.W., Bouzou, B., and Cha, J.H. (2008). Huntingtin modulates transcription, occupies gene promoters in vivo, and binds directly to DNA in a polyglutamine-dependent manner. *J. Neurosci. 28*, 10720-10733.

Bennett, E.J., Shaler, T.A., Woodman, B., Ryu, K.Y., Zaitseva, T.S., Becker, C.H., Bates, G.P., Schulman, H., and Kopito, R.R. (2007). Global changes to the ubiquitin system in Huntington's disease. *Nature 448*, 704-708.

Bett, J.S., Goellner, G.M., Woodman, B., Pratt, G., Rechsteiner, M., and Bates, G.P. (2006). Proteasome impairment does not contribute to pathogenesis in R6/2 Huntington's disease mice: exclusion of proteasome activator REGgamma as a therapeutic target. *Hum. Mol. Genet. 15*, 33-44.

Boudreau, R.L., McBride, J.L., Martins, I., Shen, S., Xing, Y., Carter, B.J., and Davidson, B.L. (2009). Nonallele-specific silencing of mutant and wild-type huntingtin demonstrates therapeutic efficacy in Huntington's disease mice. *Mol. Ther. 17*, 1053-1063.

Bowman, A.B., Yoo, S.Y., Dantuma, N.P., and Zoghbi, H.Y. (2005). Neuronal dysfunction in a polyglutamine disease model occurs in the absence of ubiquitin-proteasome system impairment and inversely correlates with the degree of nuclear inclusion formation. *Hum. Mol. Genet. 14*, 679-691.

Browne, S.E. (2008). Mitochondria and Huntington's disease pathogenesis: insight from genetic and chemical models. *Annals of the New York Academy of Sciences 1147*, 358-382.

Browne, S.E., Ferrante, R.J., and Beal, M.F. (1999). Oxidative stress in Huntington's disease. *Brain Pathol. 9*, 147-163.

Butler, D.C., McLear, J.A., and Messer, A. (2012). Engineered antibody therapies to counteract mutant huntingtin and related toxic intracellular proteins. *Prog. Neurobiol. 97*, 190-204.

Carmichael, J., Chatellier, J., Woolfson, A., Milstein, C., Fersht, A.R., and Rubinsztein, D.C. (2000). Bacterial and yeast chaperones reduce both aggregate formation and cell death in mammalian cell models of Huntington's disease. *Proceedings of the National Academy of Sciences of the United States of America 97*, 9701-9705.

Caviston, J.P., and Holzbaur, E.L. (2009). Huntingtin as an essential integrator of intracellular vesicular trafficking. *Trends in cell biology 19*, 147-155.

Cepeda, C., Ariano, M.A., Calvert, C.R., Flores-Hernandez, J., Chandler, S.H., Leavitt, B.R., Hayden, M.R., and Levine, M.S. (2001). NMDA receptor function in mouse models of Huntington disease. *J. Neurosci. Res. 66*, 525-539.

Cha, J.H. (2007). Transcriptional signatures in Huntington's disease. Prog. Neurobiol. *83*, 228-248.

Cha, J.H., Frey, A.S., Alsdorf, S.A., Kerner, J.A., Kosinski, C.M., Mangiarini, L., Penney, J.B., Jr., Davies, S.W., Bates, G.P., and Young, A.B. (1999). Altered neurotransmitter receptor expression in transgenic mouse models of Huntington's disease. *Philos Trans. R. Soc. Lond. B. Biol. Sci. 354*, 981-989.

Cha, J.H., Kosinski, C.M., Kerner, J.A., Alsdorf, S.A., Mangiarini, L., Davies, S.W., Penney, J.B., Bates, G.P., and Young, A.B. (1998). Altered brain neurotransmitter receptors in transgenic mice expressing a portion of an abnormal human huntington disease gene. *Proceedings of the National Academy of Sciences of the United States of America 95*, 6480-6485.

Chan, E.Y., Luthi-Carter, R., Strand, A., Solano, S.M., Hanson, S.A., DeJohn, M.M., Kooperberg, C., Chase, K.O., DiFiglia, M., Young, A.B., *et al.* (2002). Increased huntingtin protein length reduces the number of polyglutamine-induced gene expression changes in mouse models of Huntington's disease. *Hum. Mol. Genet. 11*, 1939-1951.

Chang, D.T., Rintoul, G.L., Pandipati, S., and Reynolds, I.J. (2006). Mutant huntingtin aggregates impair mitochondrial movement and trafficking in cortical neurons. *Neurobiol. Dis. 22*, 388-400.

Chaturvedi, R.K., Adhihetty, P., Shukla, S., Hennessy, T., Calingasan, N., Yang, L., Starkov, A., Kiaei, M., Cannella, M., Sassone, J., *et al.* (2009). Impaired PGC-1alpha function in muscle in Huntington's disease. *Hum. Mol. Genet. 18*, 3048-3065.

Che, H.V., Metzger, S., Portal, E., Deyle, C., Riess, O., and Nguyen, H.P. (2011). Localization of sequence variations in PGC-1alpha influence their modifying effect in Huntington disease. *Mol. Neurodegener 6*, 1.

Choo, Y.S., Johnson, G.V., MacDonald, M., Detloff, P.J., and Lesort, M. (2004). Mutant huntingtin directly increases susceptibility of mitochondria to the calcium-induced permeability transition and cytochrome c release. *Hum. Mol. Genet. 13*, 1407-1420.

Chopra, V., Fox, J.H., Lieberman, G., Dorsey, K., Matson, W., Waldmeier, P., Housman, D.E., Kazantsev, A., Young, A.B., and Hersch, S. (2007). A small-molecule therapeutic lead for Huntington's disease: preclinical pharmacology and efficacy of C2-8 in the R6/2 transgenic mouse. *Proceedings of the National Academy of Sciences of the United States of America 104*, 16685-16689.

Clifford, J.J., Drago, J., Natoli, A.L., Wong, J.Y., Kinsella, A., Waddington, J.L., and Vaddadi, K.S. (2002). Essential fatty acids given from conception prevent topographies of motor deficit in a transgenic model of Huntington's disease. *Neuroscience 109*, 81-88.

Colin, E., Zala, D., Liot, G., Rangone, H., Borrell-Pages, M., Li, X.J., Saudou, F., and Humbert, S. (2008). Huntingtin phosphorylation acts as a molecular switch for anterograde/retrograde transport in neurons. *EMBO J. 27*, 2124-2134.

Cong, X., Held, J.M., DeGiacomo, F., Bonner, A., Chen, J.M., Schilling, B., Czerwieniec, G.A., Gibson, B.W., and Ellerby, L.M. (2011). Mass spectrometric identification of novel lysine acetylation sites in huntingtin. *Mol. Cell. Proteomics 10*, M111 009829.

Cooper, J.K., Schilling, G., Peters, M.F., Herring, W.J., Sharp, A.H., Kaminsky, Z., Masone, J., Khan, F.A., Delanoy, M., Borchelt, D.R., *et al.* (1998). Truncated N-terminal fragments of huntingtin with expanded glutamine repeats form nuclear and cytoplasmic aggregates in cell culture. *Hum. Mol. Genet. 7*, 783-790.

Cornett, J., Cao, F., Wang, C.E., Ross, C.A., Bates, G.P., Li, S.H., and Li, X.J. (2005). Polyglutamine expansion of huntingtin impairs its nuclear export. *Nat. Genet. 37*, 198-204.

Crippa, V., Carra, S., Rusmini, P., Sau, D., Bolzoni, E., Bendotti, C., De Biasi, S., and Poletti, A. (2010). A role of small heat shock protein B8 (HspB8) in the autophagic removal of misfolded proteins responsible for neurodegenerative diseases. *Autophagy 6*, 958-960.

Cui, L., Jeong, H., Borovecki, F., Parkhurst, C.N., Tanese, N., and Krainc, D. (2006). Transcriptional repression of PGC-1alpha by mutant huntingtin leads to mitochondrial dysfunction and neurodegeneration. *Cell. 127*, 59-69.

Davies, S.W., Turmaine, M., Cozens, B.A., DiFiglia, M., Sharp, A.H., Ross, C.A., Scherzinger, E., Wanker, E.E., Mangiarini, L., and Bates, G.P. (1997). Formation of neuronal intranuclear inclusions underlies the neurological dysfunction in mice transgenic for the HD mutation. *Cell. 90*, 537-548.

Diaz-Hernandez, M., Hernandez, F., Martin-Aparicio, E., Gomez-Ramos, P., Moran, M.A., Castano, J.G., Ferrer, I., Avila, J., and Lucas, J.J. (2003). Neuronal induction of the immunoproteasome in Huntington's disease. *J. Neurosci. 23*, 11653-11661.

Diekmann, H., Anichtchik, O., Fleming, A., Futter, M., Goldsmith, P., Roach, A., and Rubinsztein, D.C. (2009). Decreased BDNF levels are a major contributor to the embryonic phenotype of huntingtin knockdown zebrafish. *J. Neurosci. 29*, 1343-1349.

DiFiglia, M. (1997). Aggregation of Huntingtin in Neuronal Intranuclear Inclusions and Dystrophic Neurites in Brain. *Science 277*, 1990-1993.

DiFiglia, M., Sapp, E., Chase, K., Schwarz, C., Meloni, A., Young, C., Martin, E., Vonsattel, J.P., Carraway, R., Reeves, S.A., *et al.* (1995). Huntingtin is a cytoplasmic protein associated with vesicles in human and rat brain neurons. *Neuron. 14*, 1075-1081.

DiFiglia, M., Sena-Esteves, M., Chase, K., Sapp, E., Pfister, E., Sass, M., Yoder, J., Reeves, P., Pandey, R.K., Rajeev, K.G., *et al.* (2007). Therapeutic silencing of mutant huntingtin with siRNA attenuates striatal and cortical neuropathology and behavioral deficits. *Proceedings of the National Academy of Sciences of the United States of America 104*, 17204-17209.

Ding, Q., Lewis, J.J., Strum, K.M., Dimayuga, E., Bruce-Keller, A.J., Dunn, J.C., and Keller, J.N. (2002). Polyglutamine expansion, protein aggregation, proteasome activity, and neural survival. *J. Biol. Chem. 277*, 13935-13942.

Dragatsis, I., Levine, M.S., and Zeitlin, S. (2000). Inactivation of Hdh in the brain and testis results in progressive neurodegeneration and sterility in mice. *Nat. Genet. 26*, 300-306.

Drouet, V., Perrin, V., Hassig, R., Dufour, N., Auregan, G., Alves, S., Bonvento, G., Brouillet, E., Luthi-Carter, R., Hantraye, P., *et al.* (2009). Sustained effects of nonallele-specific Huntingtin silencing. *Ann. Neurol. 65*, 276-285.

Dunah, A.W., Jeong, H., Griffin, A., Kim, Y.M., Standaert, D.G., Hersch, S.M., Mouradian, M.M., Young, A.B., Tanese, N., and Krainc, D. (2002). Sp1 and TAFII130 transcriptional activity disrupted in early Huntington's disease. *Science 296*, 2238-2243.

Duyao, M.P., Auerbach, A.B., Ryan, A., Persichetti, F., Barnes, G.T., McNeil, S.M., Ge, P., Vonsattel, J.P., Gusella, J.F., Joyner, A.L., *et al.* (1995). Inactivation of the mouse Huntington's disease gene homolog Hdh. *Science 269*, 407-410.

Engelender, S., Sharp, A.H., Colomer, V., Tokito, M.K., Lanahan, A., Worley, P., Holzbaur, E.L., and Ross, C.A. (1997). Huntingtin-associated protein 1 (HAP1) interacts with the p150Glued subunit of dynactin. Hu*m. Mol. Genet. 6*, 2205-2212.

Fan, M.M., and Raymond, L.A. (2007). N-methyl-D-aspartate (NMDA) receptor function and excitotoxicity in Huntington's disease. *Prog. Neurobiol. 81*, 272-293.

Ferrante, R.J., Andreassen, O.A., Dedeoglu, A., Ferrante, K.L., Jenkins, B.G., Hersch, S.M., and Beal, M.F. (2002). Therapeutic effects of coenzyme Q10 and remacemide in transgenic mouse models of Huntington's disease. *J. Neurosci. 22*, 1592-1599.

Ferrante, R.J., Andreassen, O.A., Jenkins, B.G., Dedeoglu, A., Kuemmerle, S., Kubilus, J.K., Kaddurah-Daouk, R., Hersch, S.M., and Beal, M.F. (2000). Neuroprotective effects of creatine in a transgenic mouse model of Huntington's disease. *J. Neurosci. 20*, 4389-4397.

Ferrante, R.J., Kubilus, J.K., Lee, J., Ryu, H., Beesen, A., Zucker, B., Smith, K., Kowall, N.W., Ratan, R.R., Luthi-Carter, R., *et al.* (2003). Histone deacetylase inhibition by sodium butyrate chemotherapy ameliorates the neurodegenerative phenotype in Huntington's disease mice. *J. Neurosci. 23*, 9418-9427.

Fossale, E., Wheeler, V.C., Vrbanac, V., Lebel, L.A., Teed, A., Mysore, J.S., Gusella, J.F., MacDonald, M.E., and Persichetti, F. (2002). Identification of a presymptomatic molecular phenotype in Hdh CAG knock-in mice. *Hum. Mol. Genet. 11*, 2233-2241.

Frank, S., Ondo, W., Fahn, S., Hunter, C., Oakes, D., Plumb, S., Marshall, F., Shoulson, I., Eberly, S., Walker, F., *et al.* (2008). A study of chorea after tetrabenazine withdrawal in patients with Huntington disease. *Clin. Neuropharmacol. 31*, 127-133.

Fuentealba, R.A., Marasa, J., Diamond, M.I., Piwnica-Worms, D., and Weihl, C.C. (2012). An aggregation sensing reporter identifies leflunomide and teriflunomide as polyglutamine aggregate inhibitors. *Hum. Mol. Genet. 21*, 664-680.

Fusco, F.R., Zuccato, C., Tartari, M., Martorana, A., De March, Z., Giampa, C., Cattaneo, E., and Bernardi, G. (2003). Co-localization of brain-derived neurotrophic factor (BDNF) and wild-type huntingtin in normal and quinolinic acid-lesioned rat brain. *Eur. J. Neurosci. 18*, 1093-1102.

Gafni, J., and Ellerby, L.M. (2002). Calpain activation in Huntington's disease. *J. Neurosci. 22*, 4842-4849.

Gafni, J., Hermel, E., Young, J.E., Wellington, C.L., Hayden, M.R., and Ellerby, L.M. (2004). Inhibition of calpain cleavage of huntingtin reduces toxicity: accumulation of calpain/caspase fragments in the nucleus. *J. Biol. Chem. 279*, 20211-20220.

Gardian, G., Browne, S.E., Choi, D.K., Klivenyi, P., Gregorio, J., Kubilus, J.K., Ryu, H., Langley, B., Ratan, R.R., Ferrante, R.J., *et al.* (2005). Neuroprotective effects of phenylbutyrate in the N171-82Q transgenic mouse model of Huntington's disease. *J. Biol. Chem. 280*, 556-563.

Gaughwin, P.M., Ciesla, M., Lahiri, N., Tabrizi, S.J., Brundin, P., and Bjorkqvist, M. (2011). Hsa-miR-34b is a plasma-stable microRNA that is elevated in pre-manifest Huntington's disease. *Hum. Mol. Genet. 20*, 2225-2237.

Gauthier, L.R., Charrin, B.C., Borrell-Pages, M., Dompierre, J.P., Rangone, H., Cordelieres, F.P., De Mey, J., MacDonald, M.E., Lessmann, V., Humbert, S., *et al.* (2004). Huntingtin controls neurotrophic support and survival of neurons by enhancing BDNF vesicular transport along microtubules. *Cell. 118*, 127-138.

Gervais, F.G., Singaraja, R., Xanthoudakis, S., Gutekunst, C.A., Leavitt, B.R., Metzler, M., Hackam, A.S., Tam, J., Vaillancourt, J.P., Houtzager, V., *et al.* (2002). Recruitment and activation of caspase-8 by the Huntingtin-interacting protein Hip-1 and a novel partner Hippi. *Nat. Cell. Biol. 4*, 95-105.

Ghose, J., Sinha, M., Das, E., Jana, N.R., and Bhattacharyya, N.P. (2011). Regulation of miR-146a by RelA/NFkB and p53 in STHdh(Q111)/Hdh(Q111) cells, a cell model of Huntington's disease. *PLoS One 6*, e23837.

Goffredo, D., Rigamonti, D., Tartari, M., De Micheli, A., Verderio, C., Matteoli, M., Zuccato, C., and Cattaneo, E. (2002). Calcium-dependent cleavage of endogenous wild-type huntingtin in primary cortical neurons. *J. Biol. Chem. 277*, 39594-39598.

Goldberg, Y.P., Nicholson, D.W., Rasper, D.M., Kalchman, M.A., Koide, H.B., Graham, R.K., Bromm, M., Kazemi-Esfarjani, P., Thornberry, N.A., Vaillancourt, J.P., *et al.* (1996). Cleavage of huntingtin by apopain, a proapoptotic cysteine protease, is modulated by the polyglutamine tract. *Nat. Genet. 13*, 442-449.

Graham, R.K., Deng, Y., Carroll, J., Vaid, K., Cowan, C., Pouladi, M.A., Metzler, M., Bissada, N., Wang, L., Faull, R.L., *et al.* (2010). Cleavage at the 586 amino acid caspase-6 site in mutant huntingtin influences caspase-6 activation in vivo. *J. Neurosci. 30*, 15019-15029.

Graham, R.K., Deng, Y., Slow, E.J., Haigh, B., Bissada, N., Lu, G., Pearson, J., Shehadeh, J., Bertram, L., Murphy, Z., *et al.* (2006). Cleavage at the caspase-6 site is required for neuronal dysfunction and degeneration due to mutant huntingtin. *Cell. 125*, 1179-1191.

Gray, M., Shirasaki, D.I., Cepeda, C., Andre, V.M., Wilburn, B., Lu, X.H., Tao, J., Yamazaki, I., Li, S.H., Sun, Y.E., *et al.* (2008). Full-length human mutant huntingtin with a stable polyglutamine repeat can elicit progressive and selective neuropathogenesis in BACHD mice. *J. Neurosci. 28*, 6182-6195.

Gu, X., Greiner, E.R., Mishra, R., Kodali, R., Osmand, A., Finkbeiner, S., Steffan, J.S., Thompson, L.M., Wetzel, R., and Yang, X.W. (2009). Serines 13 and 16 are critical determinants of full-length human mutant huntingtin induced disease pathogenesis in HD mice. *Neuron. 64*, 828-840.

Gunawardena, S., Her, L.S., Brusch, R.G., Laymon, R.A., Niesman, I.R., Gordesky-Gold, B., Sintasath, L., Bonini, N.M., and Goldstein, L.S. (2003). Disruption of axonal transport by loss of huntingtin or expression of pathogenic polyQ proteins in Drosophila. *Neuron. 40*, 25-40.

Gutekunst, C.A., Levey, A.I., Heilman, C.J., Whaley, W.L., Yi, H., Nash, N.R., Rees, H.D., Madden, J.J., and Hersch, S.M. (1995). Identification and localization of huntingtin in brain and human lymphoblastoid cell lines with anti-fusion protein antibodies. *Proceedings of the National Academy of Sciences of the United States of America 92*, 8710-8714.

Hackam, A.S., Singaraja, R., Wellington, C.L., Metzler, M., McCutcheon, K., Zhang, T., Kalchman, M., and Hayden, M.R. (1998). The influence of huntingtin protein size on nuclear localization and cellular toxicity. *J. Cell. Biol. 141*, 1097-1105.

Handley, O.J., Naji, J.J., Dunnett, S.B., and Rosser, A.E. (2006). Pharmaceutical, cellular and genetic therapies for Huntington's disease. *Clin. Sci.* (Lond) *110*, 73-88.

Hands, S., Sajjad, M.U., Newton, M.J., and Wyttenbach, A. (2011). In vitro and in vivo aggregation of a fragment of huntingtin protein directly causes free radical production. *J. Biol. Chem. 286*, 44512-44520.

Hansson, O., Petersen, A., Leist, M., Nicotera, P., Castilho, R.F., and Brundin, P. (1999). Transgenic mice expressing a Huntington's disease mutation are resistant to quinolinic acid-induced striatal excitotoxicity. *Proceedings of the National Academy of Sciences of the United States of America 96*, 8727-8732.

Harjes, P., and Wanker, E.E. (2003). The hunt for huntingtin function: interaction partners tell many different stories. *Trends in Biochemical Sciences 28*, 425-433.

Harper, S.Q., Staber, P.D., He, X., Eliason, S.L., Martins, I.H., Mao, Q., Yang, L., Kotin, R.M., Paulson, H.L., and Davidson, B.L. (2005). RNA interference improves motor and neuropathological abnormalities in a Huntington's disease mouse model. *Proceedings of the National Academy of Sciences of the United States of America 102*, 5820-5825.

Heiser, V., Engemann, S., Brocker, W., Dunkel, I., Boeddrich, A., Waelter, S., Nordhoff, E., Lurz, R., Schugardt, N., Rautenberg, S., *et al.* (2002). Identification of benzothiazoles as potential polyglutamine aggregation inhibitors of Huntington's disease by using an automated filter retardation assay. *Proceedings of the National Academy of Sciences of the United States of America 99 Suppl 4*, 16400-16406.

Her, L.S., and Goldstein, L.S. (2008). Enhanced sensitivity of striatal neurons to axonal transport defects induced by mutant huntingtin. *J. Neurosci. 28*, 13662-13672.

Hermel, E., Gafni, J., Propp, S.S., Leavitt, B.R., Wellington, C.L., Young, J.E., Hackam, A.S., Logvinova, A.V., Peel, A.L., Chen, S.F., *et al.* (2004). Specific caspase interactions and amplification are involved in selective neuronal vulnerability in Huntington's disease. *Cell. Death Differ. 11*, 424-438.

Hersch, S.M., Gevorkian, S., Marder, K., Moskowitz, C., Feigin, A., Cox, M., Como, P., Zimmerman, C., Lin, M., Zhang, L., *et al.* (2006). Creatine in Huntington disease is safe, tolerable, bioavailable in brain and reduces serum 8OH2'dG. *Neurology 66*, 250-252.

Ho, L.W., Brown, R., Maxwell, M., Wyttenbach, A., and Rubinsztein, D.C. (2001). Wild type Huntingtin reduces the cellular toxicity of mutant Huntingtin in mammalian cell models of Huntington's disease. *J. Med. Genet. 38*, 450-452.

Hockly, E., Richon, V.M., Woodman, B., Smith, D.L., Zhou, X., Rosa, E., Sathasivam, K., Ghazi-Noori, S., Mahal, A., Lowden, P.A., *et al.* (2003). Suberoylanilide hydroxamic acid, a histone deacetylase inhibitor, ameliorates motor deficits in a mouse model of Huntington's disease. *Proceedings of the National Academy of Sciences of the United States of America 100*, 2041-2046.

Hockly, E., Tse, J., Barker, A.L., Moolman, D.L., Beunard, J.L., Revington, A.P., Holt, K., Sunshine, S., Moffitt, H., Sathasivam, K., *et al.* (2006). Evaluation of the benzothiazole aggregation inhibitors riluzole and PGL-135 as therapeutics for Huntington's disease. *Neurobiol. Dis. 21*, 228-236.

Hodges, A., Strand, A.D., Aragaki, A.K., Kuhn, A., Sengstag, T., Hughes, G., Elliston, L.A., Hartog, C., Goldstein, D.R., Thu, D., *et al.* (2006). Regional and cellular gene expression changes in human Huntington's disease brain. *Hum. Mol. Genet. 15*, 965-977.

Hodgson, J.G., Agopyan, N., Gutekunst, C.A., Leavitt, B.R., LePiane, F., Singaraja, R., Smith, D.J., Bissada, N., McCutcheon, K., Nasir, J., *et al.* (1999). A YAC mouse model for Huntington's disease with full-length mutant huntingtin, cytoplasmic toxicity, and selective striatal neurodegeneration. *Neuron. 23*, 181-192.

Hoffner, G., Kahlem, P., and Djian, P. (2002). Perinuclear localization of huntingtin as a consequence of its binding to microtubules through an interaction with beta-tubulin: relevance to Huntington's disease. *J. Cell. Sci. 115*, 941-948.

Hogarth, P., Lovrecic, L., and Krainc, D. (2007). Sodium phenylbutyrate in Huntington's disease: a dose-finding study. Movement disorders : *official journal of the Movement Disorder Society 22*, 1962-1964.

Holmberg, C.I., Staniszewski, K.E., Mensah, K.N., Matouschek, A., and Morimoto, R.I. (2004). Inefficient degradation of truncated polyglutamine proteins by the proteasome. *EMBO J. 23*, 4307-4318.

Humbert, S., Bryson, E.A., Cordelieres, F.P., Connors, N.C., Datta, S.R., Finkbeiner, S., Greenberg, M.E., and Saudou, F. (2002). The IGF-1/Akt pathway is neuroprotective in Huntington's disease and involves Huntingtin phosphorylation by Akt. *Dev. Cell. 2*, 831-837.

Huntington Study, G. (2001). A randomized, placebo-controlled trial of coenzyme Q10 and remacemide in Huntington's disease. *Neurology 57*, 397-404.

Huntington Study, G. (2006). Tetrabenazine as antichorea therapy in Huntington disease: a randomized controlled trial. *Neurology 66*, 366-372.

Huntington Study Group, T.-H.D.I. (2008). Randomized controlled trial of ethyl-eicosapentaenoic acid in Huntington disease: the TREND-HD study. *Archives of neurology 65*, 1582-1589.

Iwata, A., Riley, B.E., Johnston, J.A., and Kopito, R.R. (2005). HDAC6 and microtubules are required for autophagic degradation of aggregated huntingtin. *J. Biol. Chem. 280*, 40282-40292.

Jana, N.R., Tanaka, M., Wang, G., and Nukina, N. (2000). Polyglutamine length-dependent interaction of Hsp40 and Hsp70 family chaperones with truncated N-terminal huntingtin: their role in suppression of aggregation and cellular toxicity. *Hum. Mol. Genet. 9*, 2009-2018.

Jana, N.R., Zemskov, E.A., Wang, G., and Nukina, N. (2001). Altered proteasomal function due to the expression of polyglutamine-expanded truncated N-terminal huntingtin induces apoptosis by caspase activation through mitochondrial cytochrome c release. *Hum. Mol. Genet. 10*, 1049-1059.

Jarabek, B.R., Yasuda, R.P., and Wolfe, B.B. (2004). Regulation of proteins affecting NMDA receptor-induced excitotoxicity in a Huntington's mouse model. *Brain: A journal of neurology 127*, 505-516.

Jenkins, B.G., Koroshetz, W.J., Beal, M.F., and Rosen, B.R. (1993). Evidence for impairment of energy metabolism in vivo in Huntington's disease using localized 1H NMR spectroscopy. *Neurology 43*, 2689-2695.

Jeong, H., Then, F., Melia, T.J., Jr., Mazzulli, J.R., Cui, L., Savas, J.N., Voisine, C., Paganetti, P., Tanese, N., Hart, A.C., *et al.* (2009). Acetylation targets mutant huntingtin to autophagosomes for degradation. *Cell. 137*, 60-72.

Jin, J., Cheng, Y., Zhang, Y., Wood, W., Peng, Q., Hutchison, E., Mattson, M.P., Becker, K.G., and Duan, W. (2012). Interrogation of brain miRNA and mRNA expression profiles reveals a molecular regulatory network that is perturbed by mutant huntingtin. *J. Neurochem. 123*, 477-490.

Johnson, R., Zuccato, C., Belyaev, N.D., Guest, D.J., Cattaneo, E., and Buckley, N.J. (2008). A microRNA-based gene dysregulation pathway in Huntington's disease. *Neurobiol. Dis. 29*, 438-445.

Kalchman, M.A., Graham, R.K., Xia, G., Koide, H.B., Hodgson, J.G., Graham, K.C., Goldberg, Y.P., Gietz, R.D., Pickart, C.M., and Hayden,

M.R. (1996). Huntingtin is ubiquitinated and interacts with a specific ubiquitin-conjugating enzyme. *J. Biol. Chem. 271*, 19385-19394.

Kalchman, M.A., Koide, H.B., McCutcheon, K., Graham, R.K., Nichol, K., Nishiyama, K., Kazemi-Esfarjani, P., Lynn, F.C., Wellington, C., Metzler, M., *et al.* (1997). HIP1, a human homologue of S. cerevisiae Sla2p, interacts with membrane-associated huntingtin in the brain. *Nat. Genet. 16*, 44-53.

Kegel, K.B., Kim, M., Sapp, E., McIntyre, C., Castano, J.G., Aronin, N., and DiFiglia, M. (2000). Huntingtin expression stimulates endosomal-lysosomal activity, endosome tubulation, and autophagy. *J. Neurosci. 20*, 7268-7278.

Kegel, K.B., Meloni, A.R., Yi, Y., Kim, Y.J., Doyle, E., Cuiffo, B.G., Sapp, E., Wang, Y., Qin, Z.H., Chen, J.D., *et al.* (2002). Huntingtin is present in the nucleus, interacts with the transcriptional corepressor C-terminal binding protein, and represses transcription. *J. Biol. Chem. 277*, 7466-7476.

Kegel, K.B., Sapp, E., Yoder, J., Cuiffo, B., Sobin, L., Kim, Y.J., Qin, Z.H., Hayden, M.R., Aronin, N., Scott, D.L., *et al.* (2005). Huntingtin associates with acidic phospholipids at the plasma membrane. *J. Biol. Chem. 280*, 36464-36473.

Khoshnan, A., Ko, J., and Patterson, P.H. (2002). Effects of intracellular expression of anti-huntingtin antibodies of various specificities on mutant huntingtin aggregation and toxicity. *Proceedings of the National Academy of Sciences of the United States of America 99*, 1002-1007.

Kieburtz, K., Feigin, A., McDermott, M., Como, P., Abwender, D., Zimmerman, C., Hickey, C., Orme, C., Claude, K., Sotack, J., *et al.* (1996). A controlled trial of remacemide hydrochloride in Huntington's disease. *Movement disorders : official journal of the Movement Disorder Society 11*, 273-277.

Kim, M., Lee, H.S., LaForet, G., McIntyre, C., Martin, E.J., Chang, P., Kim, T.W., Williams, M., Reddy, P.H., Tagle, D., *et al.* (1999). Mutant huntingtin expression in clonal striatal cells: dissociation of inclusion formation and neuronal survival by caspase inhibition. *J. Neurosci. 19*, 964-973.

Kim, M.W., Chelliah, Y., Kim, S.W., Otwinowski, Z., and Bezprozvanny, I. (2009). Secondary structure of Huntingtin amino-terminal region. *Structure 17*, 1205-1212.

Kita, H., Carmichael, J., Swartz, J., Muro, S., Wyttenbach, A., Matsubara, K., Rubinsztein, D.C., and Kato, K. (2002). Modulation of polyglutamine-induced cell death by genes identified by expression profiling. *Hum. Mol. Genet. 11*, 2279-2287.

Ko, J., Ou, S., and Patterson, P.H. (2001). New anti-huntingtin monoclonal antibodies: implications for huntingtin conformation and its binding proteins. *Brain Res. Bull 56*, 319-329.

Koga, H., Martinez-Vicente, M., Arias, E., Kaushik, S., Sulzer, D., and Cuervo, A.M. (2011). Constitutive upregulation of chaperone-mediated autophagy in Huntington's disease. *J. Neurosci. 31*, 18492-18505.

Kordasiewicz, H.B., Stanek, L.M., Wancewicz, E.V., Mazur, C., McAlonis, M.M., Pytel, K.A., Artates, J.W., Weiss, A., Cheng, S.H., Shihabuddin, L.S., *et al.* (2012). Sustained therapeutic reversal of Huntington's disease by transient repression of huntingtin synthesis. *Neuron. 74*, 1031-1044.

Kovtun, I.V., Liu, Y., Bjoras, M., Klungland, A., Wilson, S.H., and McMurray, C.T. (2007). OGG1 initiates age-dependent CAG trinucleotide expansion in somatic cells. *Nature 447*, 447-452.

Kremer, B., Clark, C.M., Almqvist, E.W., Raymond, L.A., Graf, P., Jacova, C., Mezei, M., Hardy, M.A., Snow, B., Martin, W., *et al.* (1999). Influence of lamotrigine on progression of early Huntington disease: a randomized clinical trial. *Neurology 53*, 1000-1011.

Kuemmerle, S., Gutekunst, C.A., Klein, A.M., Li, X.J., Li, S.H., Beal, M.F., Hersch, S.M., and Ferrante, R.J. (1999). Huntington aggregates may not predict neuronal death in Huntington's disease. *Ann. Neurol. 46*, 842-849.

Kuhl, D.E., Phelps, M.E., Markham, C.H., Metter, E.J., Riege, W.H., and Winter, J. (1982). Cerebral metabolism and atrophy in Huntington's disease determined by 18FDG and computed tomographic scan. *Ann. Neurol. 12*, 425-434.

Landles, C., Sathasivam, K., Weiss, A., Woodman, B., Moffitt, H., Finkbeiner, S., Sun, B., Gafni, J., Ellerby, L.M., Trottier, Y., *et al.* (2010). Proteolysis of mutant huntingtin produces an exon 1 fragment that accumulates as an aggregated protein in neuronal nuclei in Huntington disease. *J. Biol. Chem. 285*, 8808-8823.

Landwehrmeyer, G.B., Dubois, B., de Yebenes, J.G., Kremer, B., Gaus, W., Kraus, P.H., Przuntek, H., Dib, M., Doble, A., Fischer, W., *et al.* (2007). Riluzole in Huntington's disease: a 3-year, randomized controlled study. *Ann. Neurol. 62*, 262-272.

Leavitt, B.R., van Raamsdonk, J.M., Shehadeh, J., Fernandes, H., Murphy, Z., Graham, R.K., Wellington, C.L., Raymond, L.A., and Hayden, M.R. (2006). Wild-type huntingtin protects neurons from excitotoxicity. *J. Neurochem. 96*, 1121-1129.

Lecerf, J.M., Shirley, T.L., Zhu, Q., Kazantsev, A., Amersdorfer, P., Housman, D.E., Messer, A., and Huston, J.S. (2001). Human single-chain Fv intrabodies counteract in situ huntingtin aggregation in cellular models of Huntington's disease. *Proceedings of the National Academy of Sciences of the United States of America 98*, 4764-4769.

Lee, W.C., Yoshihara, M., and Littleton, J.T. (2004). Cytoplasmic aggregates trap polyglutamine-containing proteins and block axonal transport in a Drosophila model of Huntington's disease. *Proceedings of the National Academy of Sciences of the United States of America 101*, 3224-3229.

Leenders, K.L., Frackowiak, R.S., Quinn, N., and Marsden, C.D. (1986). Brain energy metabolism and dopaminergic function in Huntington's disease measured in vivo using positron emission tomography. *Movement disorders : official journal of the Movement Disorder Society 1*, 69-77.

Levine, M.S., Klapstein, G.J., Koppel, A., Gruen, E., Cepeda, C., Vargas, M.E., Jokel, E.S., Carpenter, E.M., Zanjani, H., Hurst, R.S., *et al.* (1999). Enhanced sensitivity to N-methyl-D-aspartate receptor activation in transgenic and knockin mouse models of Huntington's disease. *J. Neurosci. Res. 58*, 515-532.

Li, H., Li, S.H., Yu, Z.X., Shelbourne, P., and Li, X.J. (2001). Huntingtin aggregate-associated axonal degeneration is an early pathological event in Huntington's disease mice. *J. Neurosci. 21*, 8473-8481.

Li, S.H., Cheng, A.L., Zhou, H., Lam, S., Rao, M., Li, H., and Li, X.J. (2002a). Interaction of Huntington Disease Protein with Transcriptional Activator Sp1. *Molecular and Cellular Biology 22*, 1277-1287.

Li, S.H., Gutekunst, C.A., Hersch, S.M., and Li, X.J. (1998). Interaction of huntingtin-associated protein with dynactin P150Glued. *J. Neurosci. 18*, 1261-1269.

Li, S.H., and Li, X.J. (1998). Aggregation of N-terminal huntingtin is dependent on the length of its glutamine repeats. *Hum. Mol. Genet. 7*, 777-782.

Li, S.H., and Li, X.J. (2004). Huntingtin-protein interactions and the pathogenesis of Huntington's disease. *Trends Genet. 20*, 146-154.

Li, S.H., Schilling, G., Young, W.S., 3rd, Li, X.J., Margolis, R.L., Stine, O.C., Wagster, M.V., Abbott, M.H., Franz, M.L., Ranen, N.G., *et al.* (1993). Huntington's disease gene (IT15) is widely expressed in human and rat tissues. *Neuron. 11*, 985-993.

Li, X., Valencia, A., Sapp, E., Masso, N., Alexander, J., Reeves, P., Kegel, K.B., Aronin, N., and Difiglia, M. (2010). Aberrant Rab11-dependent trafficking of the neuronal glutamate transporter EAAC1 causes oxidative stress and cell death in Huntington's disease. *J. Neurosci. 30*, 4552-4561.

Li, X.J., Li, S.H., Sharp, A.H., Nucifora, F.C., Jr., Schilling, G., Lanahan, A., Worley, P., Snyder, S.H., and Ross, C.A. (1995). A huntingtin-associated protein enriched in brain with implications for pathology. *Nature 378*, 398-402.

Li, Y., Chin, L.S., Levey, A.I., and Li, L. (2002b). Huntingtin-associated protein 1 interacts with hepatocyte growth factor-regulated tyrosine kinase substrate and functions in endosomal trafficking. *J. Biol. Chem. 277*, 28212-28221.

Lombardi, M.S., Jaspers, L., Spronkmans, C., Gellera, C., Taroni, F., Di Maria, E., Donato, S.D., and Kaemmerer, W.F. (2009). A majority of Huntington's disease patients may be treatable by individualized allele-specific RNA interference. *Exp. Neurol. 217*, 312-319.

London, E.D., Yamamura, H.I., Bird, E.D., and Coyle, J.T. (1981). Decreased receptor-binding sites for kainic acid in brains of patients with Huntington's disease. *Biological psychiatry 16*, 155-162.

Lunkes, A., Lindenberg, K.S., Ben-Haiem, L., Weber, C., Devys, D., Landwehrmeyer, G.B., Mandel, J.L., and Trottier, Y. (2002). Proteases acting on mutant huntingtin generate cleaved products that differentially build up cytoplasmic and nuclear inclusions. *Mol. Cell. 10*, 259-269.

Luo, S., and Rubinsztein, D.C. (2009). Huntingtin promotes cell survival by preventing Pak2 cleavage. *J. Cell. Sci. 122*, 875-885.

Luo, S., Vacher, C., Davies, J.E., and Rubinsztein, D.C. (2005). Cdk5 phosphorylation of huntingtin reduces its cleavage by caspases: implications for mutant huntingtin toxicity. *J. Cell. Biol. 169*, 647-656.

Luthi-Carter, R., Hanson, S.A., Strand, A.D., Bergstrom, D.A., Chun, W., Peters, N.L., Woods, A.M., Chan, E.Y., Kooperberg, C., Krainc, D., *et al.* (2002a). Dysregulation of gene expression in the R6/2 model of polyglutamine disease: parallel changes in muscle and brain. *Hum. Mol. Genet. 11*, 1911-1926.

Luthi-Carter, R., Strand, A.D., Hanson, S.A., Kooperberg, C., Schilling, G., La Spada, A.R., Merry, D.E., Young, A.B., Ross, C.A., Borchelt, D.R., *et al.* (2002b). Polyglutamine and transcription: gene expression changes shared by DRPLA and Huntington's disease mouse models reveal context-independent effects. *Hum. Mol. Genet. 11*, 1927-1937.

Mangiarini, L., Sathasivam, K., Seller, M., Cozens, B., Harper, A., Hetherington, C., Lawton, M., Trottier, Y., Lehrach, H., Davies, S.W., *et al.* (1996). Exon 1 of the HD gene with an expanded CAG repeat is sufficient to cause a progressive neurological phenotype in transgenic mice. *Cell. 87*, 493-506.

Martindale, D., Hackam, A., Wieczorek, A., Ellerby, L., Wellington, C., McCutcheon, K., Singaraja, R., Kazemi-Esfarjani, P., Devon, R., Kim, S.U., *et al.* (1998). Length of huntingtin and its polyglutamine tract influences localization and frequency of intracellular aggregates. *Nat. Genet. 18*, 150-154.

Martinez-Vicente, M., Talloczy, Z., Wong, E., Tang, G., Koga, H., Kaushik, S., de Vries, R., Arias, E., Harris, S., Sulzer, D., *et al.* (2010). Cargo recognition failure is responsible for inefficient autophagy in Huntington's disease. *Nat. Neurosci. 13*, 567-576.

Mastroberardino, P.G., Iannicola, C., Nardacci, R., Bernassola, F., De Laurenzi, V., Melino, G., Moreno, S., Pavone, F., Oliverio, S., Fesus, L., *et al.* (2002). 'Tissue' transglutaminase ablation reduces neuronal death and prolongs survival in a mouse model of Huntington's disease. *Cell. Death Differ. 9*, 873-880.

Maynard, C.J., Bottcher, C., Ortega, Z., Smith, R., Florea, B.I., Diaz-Hernandez, M., Brundin, P., Overkleeft, H.S., Li, J.Y., Lucas, J.J., *et al.* (2009). Accumulation of ubiquitin conjugates in a polyglutamine disease model occurs without global ubiquitin/proteasome system impairment. *Proceedings of the National Academy of Sciences of the United States of America 106*, 13986-13991.

McBride, J.L., Pitzer, M.R., Boudreau, R.L., Dufour, B., Hobbs, T., Ojeda, S.R., and Davidson, B.L. (2011). Preclinical safety of RNAi-mediated HTT suppression in the rhesus macaque as a potential therapy for Huntington's disease. *Mol. Ther. 19*, 2152-2162.

Miller, J.P., Holcomb, J., Al-Ramahi, I., de Haro, M., Gafni, J., Zhang, N., Kim, E., Sanhueza, M., Torcassi, C., Kwak, S., *et al.* (2010). Matrix metalloproteinases are modifiers of huntingtin proteolysis and toxicity in Huntington's disease. *Neuron. 67*, 199-212.

Modregger, J., DiProspero, N.A., Charles, V., Tagle, D.A., and Plomann, M. (2002). PACSIN 1 interacts with huntingtin and is absent from synaptic varicosities in presymptomatic Huntington's disease brains. *Hum. Mol. Genet. 11*, 2547-2558.

Morton, A.J., and Leavens, W. (2000). Mice transgenic for the human Huntington's disease mutation have reduced sensitivity to kainic acid toxicity. *Brain Res. Bull 52*, 51-59.

Murphy, R.C., and Messer, A. (2004). A single-chain Fv intrabody provides functional protection against the effects of mutant protein in an organotypic slice culture model of Huntington's disease. *Brain Res. Mol. Brain Res. 121*, 141-145.

Nasir, J., Floresco, S.B., O'Kusky, J.R., Diewert, V.M., Richman, J.M., Zeisler, J., Borowski, A., Marth, J.D., Phillips, A.G., and Hayden, M.R. (1995). Targeted disruption of the Huntington's disease gene results in embryonic lethality and behavioral and morphological changes in heterozygotes. *Cell. 81*, 811-823.

Neveklovska, M., Clabough, E.B., Steffan, J.S., and Zeitlin, S.O. (2012). Deletion of the huntingtin proline-rich region does not significantly affect normal huntingtin function in mice. *J. Huntingtons Dis. 1*, 71-87.

Norris, P.J., Waldvogel, H.J., Faull, R.L., Love, D.R., and Emson, P.C. (1996). Decreased neuronal nitric oxide synthase messenger RNA and somatostatin messenger RNA in the striatum of Huntington's disease. *Neuroscience 72*, 1037-1047.

Novak, M.J., and Tabrizi, S.J. (2011). Huntington's disease: clinical presentation and treatment. *International review of neurobiology 98*, 297-323.

Nucifora, F.C., Jr., Sasaki, M., Peters, M.F., Huang, H., Cooper, J.K., Yamada, M., Takahashi, H., Tsuji, S., Troncoso, J., Dawson, V.L., *et al.* (2001). Interference by huntingtin and atrophin-1 with cbp-mediated transcription leading to cellular toxicity. *Science 291*, 2423-2428.

Oliveira, J.M., Chen, S., Almeida, S., Riley, R., Goncalves, J., Oliveira, C.R., Hayden, M.R., Nicholls, D.G., Ellerby, L.M., and Rego, A.C. (2006). Mitochondrial-dependent Ca2+ handling in Huntington's disease striatal cells: effect of histone deacetylase inhibitors. *J. Neurosci. 26*, 11174-11186.

Ondo, W.G., Mejia, N.I., and Hunter, C.B. (2007). A pilot study of the clinical efficacy and safety of memantine for Huntington's disease. *Parkinsonism and related disorders 13*, 453-454.

Packer, A.N., Xing, Y., Harper, S.Q., Jones, L., and Davidson, B.L. (2008). The bifunctional microRNA miR-9/miR-9* regulates REST and CoREST and is downregulated in Huntington's disease. *J. Neurosci. 28*, 14341-14346.

Panov, A.V., Burke, J.R., Strittmatter, W.J., and Greenamyre, J.T. (2003). In vitro effects of polyglutamine tracts on Ca2+-dependent depolarization of rat and human mitochondria: relevance to Huntington's disease. *Arch. Biochem. Biophys. 410*, 1-6.

Panov, A.V., Gutekunst, C.A., Leavitt, B.R., Hayden, M.R., Burke, J.R., Strittmatter, W.J., and Greenamyre, J.T. (2002). Early mitochondrial calcium defects in Huntington's disease are a direct effect of polyglutamines. *Nat. Neurosci. 5*, 731-736.

Pardo, R., Colin, E., Regulier, E., Aebischer, P., Deglon, N., Humbert, S., and Saudou, F. (2006). Inhibition of calcineurin by FK506 protects against polyglutamine-huntingtin toxicity through an increase of huntingtin phosphorylation at S421. *J. Neurosci. 26*, 1635-1645.

Parker, J.A., Connolly, J.B., Wellington, C., Hayden, M., Dausset, J., and Neri, C. (2001). Expanded polyglutamines in Caenorhabditis elegans cause axonal abnormalities and severe dysfunction of PLM mechanosensory neurons without cell death. *Proceedings of the National Academy of Sciences of the United States of America 98*, 13318-13323.

Pennuto, M., Palazzolo, I., and Poletti, A. (2009). Post-translational modifications of expanded polyglutamine proteins: impact on neurotoxicity. *Hum. Mol. Genet. 18*, R40-47.

Peters, M.F., and Ross, C.A. (2001). Isolation of a 40-kDa Huntingtin-associated protein. *J. Biol. Chem. 276*, 3188-3194.

Petersen, A., Larsen, K.E., Behr, G.G., Romero, N., Przedborski, S., Brundin, P., and Sulzer, D. (2001). Expanded CAG repeats in exon 1 of the Huntington's disease gene stimulate dopamine-mediated striatal neuron autophagy and degeneration. *Hum. Mol. Genet. 10*, 1243-1254.

Pfister, E.L., Kennington, L., Straubhaar, J., Wagh, S., Liu, W., DiFiglia, M., Landwehrmeyer, B., Vonsattel, J.P., Zamore, P.D., and Aronin, N. (2009). Five siRNAs targeting three SNPs may provide therapy for three-quarters of Huntington's disease patients. *Curr. Biol. 19*, 774-778.

Puri, B.K., Bydder, G.M., Counsell, S.J., Corridan, B.J., Richardson, A.J., Hajnal, J.V., Appel, C., McKee, H.M., Vaddadi, K.S., and Horrobin, D.F. (2002). MRI and neuropsychological improvement in Huntington disease following ethyl-EPA treatment. *Neuroreport 13*, 123-126.

Puri, B.K., Leavitt, B.R., Hayden, M.R., Ross, C.A., Rosenblatt, A., Greenamyre, J.T., Hersch, S., Vaddadi, K.S., Sword, A., Horrobin, D.F., *et al.* (2005). Ethyl-EPA in Huntington disease: a double-blind, randomized, placebo-controlled trial. *Neurology 65*, 286-292.

Qin, Z.H., Wang, Y., Kegel, K.B., Kazantsev, A., Apostol, B.L., Thompson, L.M., Yoder, J., Aronin, N., and DiFiglia, M. (2003). Autophagy regulates the processing of amino terminal huntingtin fragments. *Hum. Mol. Genet. 12*, 3231-3244.

Ratovitski, T., Nakamura, M., D'Ambola, J., Chighladze, E., Liang, Y., Wang, W., Graham, R., Hayden, M.R., Borchelt, D.R., Hirschhorn, R.R., *et al.* (2007). N-terminal proteolysis of full-length mutant huntingtin in an inducible PC12 cell model of Huntington's disease. *Cell. Cycle 6*, 2970-2981.

Ravikumar, B., Duden, R., and Rubinsztein, D.C. (2002). Aggregate-prone proteins with polyglutamine and polyalanine expansions are degraded by autophagy. *Hum. Mol. Genet. 11*, 1107-1117.

Ravikumar, B., Vacher, C., Berger, Z., Davies, J.E., Luo, S., Oroz, L.G., Scaravilli, F., Easton, D.F., Duden, R., O'Kane, C.J., *et al.* (2004). Inhibition of mTOR induces autophagy and reduces toxicity of polyglutamine expansions in fly and mouse models of Huntington disease. *Nat. Genet. 36*, 585-595.

Rigamonti, D., Bauer, J.H., De-Fraja, C., Conti, L., Sipione, S., Sciorati, C., Clementi, E., Hackam, A., Hayden, M.R., Li, Y., *et al.* (2000). Wild-type huntingtin protects from apoptosis upstream of caspase-3. *J. Neurosci. 20*, 3705-3713.

Rigamonti, D., Sipione, S., Goffredo, D., Zuccato, C., Fossale, E., and Cattaneo, E. (2001). Huntingtin's neuroprotective activity occurs via inhibition of procaspase-9 processing. *J. Biol. Chem. 276*, 14545-14548.

Rockabrand, E., Slepko, N., Pantalone, A., Nukala, V.N., Kazantsev, A., Marsh, J.L., Sullivan, P.G., Steffan, J.S., Sensi, S.L., and Thompson, L.M. (2007). The first 17 amino acids of Huntingtin modulate its sub-cellular localization, aggregation and effects on calcium homeostasis. *Hum. Mol. Genet. 16*, 61-77.

Roizin, L., Stellar, S., Willson, N., Whittier, J., and Liu, J.C. (1974). Electron microscope and enzyme studies in cerebral biopsies of Huntington's chorea. *Trans Am. Neurol. Assoc. 99*, 240-243.

Rosas, H.D., Hevelone, N.D., Zaleta, A.K., Greve, D.N., Salat, D.H., and Fischl, B. (2005). Regional cortical thinning in preclinical Huntington disease and its relationship to cognition. *Neurology 65*, 745-747.

Rosas, H.D., Koroshetz, W.J., Chen, Y.I., Skeuse, C., Vangel, M., Cudkowicz, M.E., Caplan, K., Marek, K., Seidman, L.J., Makris, N., *et al.* (2003). Evidence for more widespread cerebral pathology in early HD: an MRI-based morphometric analysis. *Neurology 60*, 1615-1620.

Rosas, H.D., Koroshetz, W.J., Jenkins, B.G., Chen, Y.I., Hayden, D.L., Beal, M.F., and Cudkowicz, M.E. (1999). Riluzole therapy in Huntington's disease (HD). *Movement disorders : official journal of the Movement Disorder Society 14*, 326-330.

Rosas, H.D., Salat, D.H., Lee, S.Y., Zaleta, A.K., Pappu, V., Fischl, B., Greve, D., Hevelone, N., and Hersch, S.M. (2008). Cerebral cortex and the clinical expression of Huntington's disease: complexity and heterogeneity. *Brain : a journal of neurology 131*, 1057-1068.

Rose, C., Menzies, F.M., Renna, M., Acevedo-Arozena, A., Corrochano, S., Sadiq, O., Brown, S.D., and Rubinsztein, D.C. (2010). Rilmenidine attenuates toxicity of polyglutamine expansions in a mouse model of Huntington's disease. *Hum. Mol. Genet. 19*, 2144-2153.

Ross, C.A. (2002). Polyglutamine pathogenesis: emergence of unifying mechanisms for Huntington's disease and related disorders. *Neuron 35*, 819-822.

Ruan, Q., Quintanilla, R.A., and Johnson, G.V. (2007). Type 2 transglutaminase differentially modulates striatal cell death in the presence of wild type or mutant huntingtin. *J. Neurochem. 102*, 25-36.

Sah, D.W., and Aronin, N. (2011). Oligonucleotide therapeutic approaches for Huntington disease. *J. Clin. Invest. 121*, 500-507.

Sanberg, P.R., Calderon, S.F., Giordano, M., Tew, J.M., and Norman, A.B. (1989). The quinolinic acid model of Huntington's disease: locomotor abnormalities. *Exp. Neurol. 105*, 45-53.

Sanchez, I., Mahlke, C., and Yuan, J. (2003). Pivotal role of oligomerization in expanded polyglutamine neurodegenerative disorders. *Nature 421*, 373-379.

Sarkar, S., Davies, J.E., Huang, Z., Tunnacliffe, A., and Rubinsztein, D.C. (2007). Trehalose, a novel mTOR-independent autophagy enhancer, accelerates the clearance of mutant huntingtin and alpha-synuclein. *J. Biol. Chem. 282*, 5641-5652.

Sarkar, S., Floto, R.A., Berger, Z., Imarisio, S., Cordenier, A., Pasco, M., Cook, L.J., and Rubinsztein, D.C. (2005). Lithium induces autophagy by inhibiting inositol monophosphatase. *J. Cell. Biol. 170*, 1101-1111.

Sarkar, S., Krishna, G., Imarisio, S., Saiki, S., O'Kane, C.J., and Rubinsztein, D.C. (2008). A rational mechanism for combination treatment of Huntington's disease using lithium and rapamycin. *Hum. Mol. Genet. 17*, 170-178.

Sarkar, S., and Rubinsztein, D.C. (2008). Huntington's disease: degradation of mutant huntingtin by autophagy. *FEBS J. 275*, 4263-4270.

Schiefer, J., Landwehrmeyer, G.B., Luesse, H.G., Sprunken, A., Puls, C., Milkereit, A., Milkereit, E., and Kosinski, C.M. (2002). Riluzole prolongs survival time and alters nuclear inclusion formation in a transgenic mouse model of Huntington's disease. *Movement disorders : official journal of the Movement Disorder Society 17*, 748-757.

Schilling, G., Coonfield, M.L., Ross, C.A., and Borchelt, D.R. (2001). Coenzyme Q10 and remacemide hydrochloride ameliorate motor deficits in a Huntington's disease transgenic mouse model. *Neurosci. Lett. 315*, 149-153.

Schwarcz, R., Foster, A.C., French, E.D., Whetsell, W.O., Jr., and Kohler, C. (1984). Excitotoxic models for neurodegenerative disorders. *Life sciences 35*, 19-32.

Seo, H., Kim, W., and Isacson, O. (2008). Compensatory changes in the ubiquitin-proteasome system, brain-derived neurotrophic factor and mitochondrial complex II/III in YAC72 and R6/2 transgenic mice partially model Huntington's disease patients. *Hum. Mol. Genet. 17*, 3144-3153.

Seo, H., Sonntag, K.C., and Isacson, O. (2004). Generalized brain and skin proteasome inhibition in Huntington's disease. *Ann. Neurol. 56*, 319-328.

Seppi, K., Mueller, J., Bodner, T., Brandauer, E., Benke, T., Weirich-Schwaiger, H., Poewe, W., and Wenning, G.K. (2001). Riluzole in Huntington's disease (HD): an open label study with one year follow up. *Journal of neurology 248*, 866-869.

Singaraja, R.R., Hadano, S., Metzler, M., Givan, S., Wellington, C.L., Warby, S., Yanai, A., Gutekunst, C.A., Leavitt, B.R., Yi, H., *et al.* (2002). HIP14, a novel ankyrin domain-containing protein, links huntingtin to intracellular trafficking and endocytosis. *Hum. Mol. Genet. 11*, 2815-2828.

Sipione, S., Rigamonti, D., Valenza, M., Zuccato, C., Conti, L., Pritchard, J., Kooperberg, C., Olson, J.M., and Cattaneo, E. (2002). Early transcriptional profiles in huntingtin-inducible striatal cells by microarray analyses. *Hum. Mol. Genet. 11*, 1953-1965.

Sittler, A., Walter, S., Wedemeyer, N., Hasenbank, R., Scherzinger, E., Eickhoff, H., Bates, G.P., Lehrach, H., and Wanker, E.E. (1998). SH3GL3 associates with the Huntingtin exon 1 protein and promotes the formation of polygln-containing protein aggregates. *Mol. Cell. 2*, 427-436.

Slow, E.J., Graham, R.K., Osmand, A.P., Devon, R.S., Lu, G., Deng, Y., Pearson, J., Vaid, K., Bissada, N., Wetzel, R., *et al.* (2005). Absence of behavioral abnormalities and neurodegeneration in vivo despite widespread neuronal huntingtin inclusions. *Proceedings of the National Academy of Sciences of the United States of America 102*, 11402-11407.

Snyder-Keller, A., McLear, J.A., Hathorn, T., and Messer, A. (2010). Early or late-stage anti-N-terminal Huntingtin intrabody gene therapy reduces pathological features in B6.HDR6/1 mice. *J. Neuropathol. Exp. Neurol. 69*, 1078-1085.

Sontag, E.M., Lotz, G.P., Agrawal, N., Tran, A., Aron, R., Yang, G., Necula, M., Lau, A., Finkbeiner, S., Glabe, C., *et al.* (2012). Methylene blue modulates huntingtin aggregation intermediates and is protective in Huntington's disease models. *J. Neurosci. 32*, 11109-11119.

Southwell, A.L., Khoshnan, A., Dunn, D.E., Bugg, C.W., Lo, D.C., and Patterson, P.H. (2008). Intrabodies binding the proline-rich domains of mutant huntingtin increase its turnover and reduce neurotoxicity. *J. Neurosci. 28*, 9013-9020.

Southwell, A.L., Ko, J., and Patterson, P.H. (2009). Intrabody gene therapy ameliorates motor, cognitive, and neuropathological symptoms in multiple mouse models of Huntington's disease. *J. Neurosci. 29*, 13589-13602.

Steffan, J.S., Agrawal, N., Pallos, J., Rockabrand, E., Trotman, L.C., Slepko, N., Illes, K., Lukacsovich, T., Zhu, Y.Z., Cattaneo, E., *et al.* (2004). SUMO modification of Huntingtin and Huntington's disease pathology. *Science 304*, 100-104.

Steffan, J.S., Bodai, L., Pallos, J., Poelman, M., McCampbell, A., Apostol, B.L., Kazantsev, A., Schmidt, E., Zhu, Y.Z., Greenwald, M., *et al.* (2001). Histone deacetylase inhibitors arrest polyglutamine-dependent neurodegeneration in Drosophila. *Nature 413*, 739-743.

Steffan, J.S., Kazantsev, A., Spasic-Boskovic, O., Greenwald, M., Zhu, Y.Z., Gohler, H., Wanker, E.E., Bates, G.P., Housman, D.E., and Thompson, L.M. (2000). The Huntington's disease protein interacts with p53 and CREB-binding protein and represses transcription. *Proceedings of the National Academy of Sciences of the United States of America 97*, 6763-6768.

Strong, T.V., Tagle, D.A., Valdes, J.M., Elmer, L.W., Boehm, K., Swaroop, M., Kaatz, K.W., Collins, F.S., and Albin, R.L. (1993). Widespread expression of the human and rat Huntington's disease gene in brain and nonneural tissues. *Nat. Genet. 5*, 259-265.

Su, S., Jou, S., Cheng, W., Lin, T., Li, J., Huang, C., Lee, Y., Soong, B., and Liu, C. (2010). Mitochondrial DNA damage in spinal and bulbar muscular atrophy patients and carriers. *Clin. Chim. Acta. 411*, 626-630.

Sugars, K.L., Brown, R., Cook, L.J., Swartz, J., and Rubinsztein, D.C. (2004). Decreased cAMP response element-mediated transcription: an early event in exon 1 and full-length cell models of Huntington's disease that contributes to polyglutamine pathogenesis. *J. Biol. Chem. 279*, 4988-4999.

Sun, Y., Savanenin, A., Reddy, P.H., and Liu, Y.F. (2001). Polyglutamine-expanded huntingtin promotes sensitization of N-methyl-D-aspartate receptors via post-synaptic density 95. *J. Biol. Chem. 276*, 24713-24718.

Tabrizi, S.J., Blamire, A.M., Manners, D.N., Rajagopalan, B., Styles, P., Schapira, A.H., and Warner, T.T. (2005). High-dose creatine therapy for Huntington disease: a 2-year clinical and MRS study. *Neurology 64*, 1655-1656.

Tanaka, M., Machida, Y., Niu, S., Ikeda, T., Jana, N.R., Doi, H., Kurosawa, M., Nekooki, M., and Nukina, N. (2004). Trehalose alleviates polyglutamine-mediated pathology in a mouse model of Huntington disease. *Nat. Med. 10*, 148-154.

Tanaka, Y., Igarashi, S., Nakamura, M., Gafni, J., Torcassi, C., Schilling, G., Crippen, D., Wood, J.D., Sawa, A., Jenkins, N.A., *et al.* (2006). Progressive phenotype and nuclear accumulation of an amino-terminal cleavage fragment in a transgenic mouse model with inducible expression of full-length mutant huntingtin. *Neurobiol.* Dis. *21*, 381-391.

Tang, T.S., Chen, X., Liu, J., and Bezprozvanny, I. (2007). Dopaminergic signaling and striatal neurodegeneration in Huntington's disease. *J. Neurosci. 27*, 7899-7910.

Tartari, M., Gissi, C., Lo Sardo, V., Zuccato, C., Picardi, E., Pesole, G., and Cattaneo, E. (2008). Phylogenetic comparison of huntingtin homologues reveals the appearance of a primitive polyQ in sea urchin. *Mol. Biol. Evol. 25*, 330-338.

Thomas, E.A., Coppola, G., Desplats, P.A., Tang, B., Soragni, E., Burnett, R., Gao, F., Fitzgerald, K.M., Borok, J.F., Herman, D., *et al.* (2008). The HDAC inhibitor 4b ameliorates the disease phenotype and transcriptional abnormalities in Huntington's disease transgenic mice. *Proceedings of the National Academy of Sciences of the United States of America 105*, 15564-15569.

Thompson, L.M., Aiken, C.T., Kaltenbach, L.S., Agrawal, N., Illes, K., Khoshnan, A., Martinez-Vincente, M., Arrasate, M., O'Rourke, J.G., Khashwji, H., *et al.* (2009). IKK phosphorylates Huntingtin and targets it for degradation by the proteasome and lysosome. *J. Cell. Biol. 187*, 1083-1099.

Truant, R., Atwal, R., and Burtnik, A. (2006). Hypothesis: Huntingtin may function in membrane association and vesicular trafficking. *Biochem.* Cell. Biol. *84*, 912-917.

Trushina, E., Dyer, R.B., Badger, J.D., 2nd, Ure, D., Eide, L., Tran, D.D., Vrieze, B.T., Legendre-Guillemin, V., McPherson, P.S., Mandavilli, B.S., *et al.* (2004). Mutant huntingtin impairs axonal trafficking in mammalian neurons in vivo and in vitro. *Mol. Cell. Biol. 24*, 8195-8209.

Tsvetkov, A.S., Miller, J., Arrasate, M., Wong, J.S., Pleiss, M.A., and Finkbeiner, S. (2010). A small-molecule scaffold induces autophagy in primary neurons and protects against toxicity in a Huntington disease model. *Proceedings of the National Academy of Sciences of the United States of America 107*, 16982-16987.

Vacher, C., Garcia-Oroz, L., and Rubinsztein, D.C. (2005). Overexpression of yeast hsp104 reduces polyglutamine aggregation and prolongs survival of a transgenic mouse model of Huntington's disease. *Hum. Mol. Genet. 14*, 3425-3433.

Valenza, M., Rigamonti, D., Goffredo, D., Zuccato, C., Fenu, S., Jamot, L., Strand, A., Tarditi, A., Woodman, B., Racchi, M., *et al.* (2005). Dysfunction of the cholesterol biosynthetic pathway in Huntington's disease. *J. Neurosci. 25*, 9932-9939.

van Bilsen, P.H., Jaspers, L., Lombardi, M.S., Odekerken, J.C., Burright, E.N., and Kaemmerer, W.F. (2008). Identification and allele-specific silencing of the mutant huntingtin allele in Huntington's disease patient-derived fibroblasts. *Hum. Gene. Ther. 19*, 710-719.

Van Raamsdonk, J.M., Pearson, J., Rogers, D.A., Lu, G., Barakauskas, V.E., Barr, A.M., Honer, W.G., Hayden, M.R., and Leavitt, B.R. (2005). Ethyl-EPA treatment improves motor dysfunction, but not neurodegeneration in the YAC128 mouse model of Huntington disease. *Exp. Neurol. 196*, 266-272.

Velier, J., Kim, M., Schwarz, C., Kim, T.W., Sapp, E., Chase, K., Aronin, N., and DiFiglia, M. (1998). Wild-type and mutant huntingtins function in vesicle trafficking in the secretory and endocytic pathways. *Exp. Neurol. 152*, 34-40.

Venkatraman, P., Wetzel, R., Tanaka, M., Nukina, N., and Goldberg, A.L. (2004). Eukaryotic proteasomes cannot digest polyglutamine sequences and release them during degradation of polyglutamine-containing proteins. *Mol. Cell. 14*, 95-104.

Waelter, S., Boeddrich, A., Lurz, R., Scherzinger, E., Lueder, G., Lehrach, H., and Wanker, E.E. (2001). Accumulation of mutant huntingtin fragments in aggresome-like inclusion bodies as a result of insufficient protein degradation. *Mol. Biol. Cell. 12*, 1393-1407.

Waldron-Roby, E., Ratovitski, T., Wang, X., Jiang, M., Watkin, E., Arbez, N., Graham, R.K., Hayden, M.R., Hou, Z., Mori, S., *et al.* (2012). Transgenic mouse model expressing the caspase 6 fragment of mutant huntingtin. *J. Neurosci. 32*, 183-193.

Wang, H., Chen, X., Li, Y., Tang, T.S., and Bezprozvanny, I. (2010). Tetrabenazine is neuroprotective in Huntington's disease mice. *Mol. Neurodegener. 5*, 18.

Wang, J., Wang, C.E., Orr, A., Tydlacka, S., Li, S.H., and Li, X.J. (2008). Impaired ubiquitin-proteasome system activity in the synapses of Huntington's disease mice. *J. Cell. Biol. 180*, 1177-1189.

Warby, S.C., Chan, E.Y., Metzler, M., Gan, L., Singaraja, R.R., Crocker, S.F., Robertson, H.A., and Hayden, M.R. (2005). Huntingtin phosphorylation on serine 421 is significantly reduced in the striatum and by polyglutamine expansion in vivo. *Hum. Mol. Genet. 14*, 1569-1577.

Warby, S.C., Montpetit, A., Hayden, A.R., Carroll, J.B., Butland, S.L., Visscher, H., Collins, J.A., Semaka, A., Hudson, T.J., and Hayden, M.R. (2009). CAG expansion in the Huntington disease gene is associated with a specific and targetable predisposing haplogroup. *Am. J. Hum. Genet. 84*, 351-366.

Warrick, J.M., Chan, H.Y., Gray-Board, G.L., Chai, Y., Paulson, H.L., and Bonini, N.M. (1999). Suppression of polyglutamine-mediated neurodegeneration in Drosophila by the molecular chaperone HSP70. *Nat. Genet. 23*, 425-428.

Wellington, C.L., Ellerby, L.M., Hackam, A.S., Margolis, R.L., Trifiro, M.A., Singaraja, R., McCutcheon, K., Salvesen, G.S., Propp, S.S., Bromm, M., *et al.* (1998). Caspase cleavage of gene products associated with triplet expansion disorders generates truncated fragments containing the polyglutamine tract. *J. Biol. Chem. 273*, 9158-9167.

Wellington, C.L., and Hayden, M.R. (2000). Caspases and neurodegeneration: on the cutting edge of new therapeutic approaches. *Clin. Genet. 57*, 1-10.

Wellington, C.L., Singaraja, R., Ellerby, L., Savill, J., Roy, S., Leavitt, B., Cattaneo, E., Hackam, A., Sharp, A., Thornberry, N., *et al.* (2000). Inhibiting caspase cleavage of huntingtin reduces toxicity and aggregate formation in neuronal and nonneuronal cells. *J. Biol. Chem. 275*, 19831-19838.

Weydt, P., Pineda, V.V., Torrence, A.E., Libby, R.T., Satterfield, T.F., Lazarowski, E.R., Gilbert, M.L., Morton, G.J., Bammler, T.K., Strand, A.D., *et al.* (2006). Thermoregulatory and metabolic defects in Huntington's disease transgenic mice implicate PGC-1alpha in Huntington's disease neurodegeneration. *Cell. Metab. 4*, 349-362.

Weydt, P., Soyal, S.M., Gellera, C., Didonato, S., Weidinger, C., Oberkofler, H., Landwehrmeyer, G.B., and Patsch, W. (2009). The gene coding for

PGC-1alpha modifies age at onset in Huntington's Disease. *Mol. Neurodegener. 4*, 3.

Williams, A., Sarkar, S., Cuddon, P., Ttofi, E.K., Saiki, S., Siddiqi, F.H., Jahreiss, L., Fleming, A., Pask, D., Goldsmith, P., *et al.* (2008). Novel targets for Huntington's disease in an mTOR-independent autophagy pathway. *Nat. Chem. Biol. 4*, 295-305.

Wolfgang, W.J., Miller, T.W., Webster, J.M., Huston, J.S., Thompson, L.M., Marsh, J.L., and Messer, A. (2005). Suppression of Huntington's disease pathology in Drosophila by human single-chain Fv antibodies. *Proceedings of the National Academy of Sciences of the United States of America 102*, 11563-11568.

Wyttenbach, A., Carmichael, J., Swartz, J., Furlong, R.A., Narain, Y., Rankin, J., and Rubinsztein, D.C. (2000). Effects of heat shock, heat shock protein 40 (HDJ-2), and proteasome inhibition on protein aggregation in cellular models of Huntington's disease. *Proceedings of the National Academy of Sciences of the United States of America 97*, 2898-2903.

Wyttenbach, A., Sauvageot, O., Carmichael, J., Diaz-Latoud, C., Arrigo, A.P., and Rubinsztein, D.C. (2002). Heat shock protein 27 prevents cellular polyglutamine toxicity and suppresses the increase of reactive oxygen species caused by huntingtin. *Hum. Mol. Genet. 11*, 1137-1151.

Wyttenbach, A., Swartz, J., Kita, H., Thykjaer, T., Carmichael, J., Bradley, J., Brown, R., Maxwell, M., Schapira, A., Orntoft, T.F., *et al.* (2001). Polyglutamine expansions cause decreased CRE-mediated transcription and early gene expression changes prior to cell death in an inducible cell model of Huntington's disease. *Hum. Mol. Genet. 10*, 1829-1845.

Yamamoto, A., Lucas, J.J., and Hen, R. (2000). Reversal of Neuropathology and Motor Dysfunction in a Conditional Model of Huntington's Disease. *Cell. 101*, 57-66.

Yanai, A., Huang, K., Kang, R., Singaraja, R.R., Arstikaitis, P., Gan, L., Orban, P.C., Mullard, A., Cowan, C.M., Raymond, L.A., *et al.* (2006). Palmitoylation of huntingtin by HIP14 is essential for its trafficking and function. *Nat. Neurosci. 9*, 824-831.

Young, A.B., Greenamyre, J.T., Hollingsworth, Z., Albin, R., D'Amato, C., Shoulson, I., and Penney, J.B. (1988). NMDA receptor losses in putamen from patients with Huntington's disease. *Science 241*, 981-983.

Yu, D., Pendergraff, H., Liu, J., Kordasiewicz, H.B., Cleveland, D.W., Swayze, E.E., Lima, W.F., Crooke, S.T., Prakash, T.P., and Corey, D.R. (2012). Single-stranded RNAs use RNAi to potently and allele-selectively inhibit mutant huntingtin expression. *Cell. 150*, 895-908.

Zala, D., Colin, E., Rangone, H., Liot, G., Humbert, S., and Saudou, F. (2008). Phosphorylation of mutant huntingtin at S421 restores anterograde and retrograde transport in neurons. *Hum. Mol. Genet. 17*, 3837-3846.

Zeitlin, S., Liu, J.P., Chapman, D.L., Papaioannou, V.E., and Efstratiadis, A. (1995). Increased apoptosis and early embryonic lethality in mice nullizygous for the Huntington's disease gene homologue. *Nat. Genet. 11*, 155-163.

Zeron, M.M., Fernandes, H.B., Krebs, C., Shehadeh, J., Wellington, C.L., Leavitt, B.R., Baimbridge, K.G., Hayden, M.R., and Raymond, L.A. (2004). Potentiation of NMDA receptor-mediated excitotoxicity linked with intrinsic apoptotic pathway in YAC transgenic mouse model of Huntington's disease. *Mol. Cell. Neurosci. 25*, 469-479.

Zeron, M.M., Hansson, O., Chen, N., Wellington, C.L., Leavitt, B.R., Brundin, P., Hayden, M.R., and Raymond, L.A. (2002). Increased sensitivity to N-methyl-D-aspartate receptor-mediated excitotoxicity in a mouse model of Huntington's disease. *Neuron. 33*, 849-860.

Zhai, W., Jeong, H., Cui, L., Krainc, D., and Tjian, R. (2005). In vitro analysis of huntingtin-mediated transcriptional repression reveals multiple transcription factor targets. *Cell. 123*, 1241-1253.

Zhang, X., Smith, D.L., Meriin, A.B., Engemann, S., Russel, D.E., Roark, M., Washington, S.L., Maxwell, M.M., Marsh, J.L., Thompson, L.M., *et al.* (2005). A potent small molecule inhibits polyglutamine aggregation in Huntington's disease neurons and suppresses neurodegeneration in vivo. *Proceedings of the National Academy of Sciences of the United States of America 102*, 892-897.

Zuccato, C., Belyaev, N., Conforti, P., Ooi, L., Tartari, M., Papadimou, E., MacDonald, M., Fossale, E., Zeitlin, S., Buckley, N., *et al.* (2007). Widespread disruption of repressor element-1 silencing transcription factor/neuron-restrictive silencer factor occupancy at its target genes in Huntington's disease. *J. Neurosci. 27*, 6972-6983.

Zuccato, C., and Cattaneo, E. (2009). Brain-derived neurotrophic factor in neurodegenerative diseases. *Nat. Rev. Neurol. 5*, 311-322.

Zuccato, C., Ciammola, A., Rigamonti, D., Leavitt, B.R., Goffredo, D., Conti, L., MacDonald, M.E., Friedlander, R.M., Silani, V., Hayden, M.R., *et al.* (2001). Loss of huntingtin-mediated BDNF gene transcription in Huntington's disease. *Science 293*, 493-498.

Zuccato, C., Tartari, M., Crotti, A., Goffredo, D., Valenza, M., Conti, L., Cataudella, T., Leavitt, B.R., Hayden, M.R., Timmusk, T., *et al.* (2003).

Huntingtin interacts with REST/NRSF to modulate the transcription of NRSE-controlled neuronal genes. *Nat. Genet. 35*, 76-83.

In: Huntington's Disease
Editors: K. Guillory, A. M. Carrasco
ISBN: 978-1-62808-316-3

Chapter II

The Role of Brain-Derived Neurotrophic Factor (BDNF) in Huntington's Disease: Trophic Support as a Therapeutic Strategy

***Patricia S. Brocardo*[1,2] *and Joana Gil-Mohapel*[1,*]**
[1]Division of Medical Sciences, Island Medical Program,
University of Victoria, Victoria, British Columbia, Canada;
[2]Neuroscience Program, Federal University of Santa Catarina,
Florianópolis, Santa Catarina, Brazil

Abstract

Huntington's disease (HD) is the most common polyglutamine neurodegenerative disorder and is caused by a mutation of an unstable expansion of CAG repeats within the coding region of the *HD* gene, which expresses the protein huntingtin. Although the abnormal protein is ubiquitously expressed throughout the organism, cell degeneration occurs

* Corresponding Author: Dr. Joana Gil-Mohapel (Ph.D.), Division of Medical Sciences, Island Medical Program, University of Victoria, Victoria, B.C., V8W 2Y2, Canada. E-mail: jgil@uvic.ca; Phone: +1.250-721-6586; Fax: +1.250-472-5505.

mainly in the brain, particularly in the striatum and cortex. The first symptoms usually appear in mid-life and include cognitive deficits and motor disturbances associated with the loss of voluntary movement coordination, which progress over time. The disease is invariably fatal and there is currently no cure for affected individuals. Although the function of normal huntingtin is still under debate, it is now known that this protein can promote the expression of the neurotrophin brain-derived neurotrophic factor (BDNF), as well as its vesicular transport along the microtubules. On the other hand, mutant huntingtin appears to impair both the neuronal expression and transport of this neurotrophic factor, thus contributing to a loss of neurotrophic support in the HD brain. In agreement with this idea, BDNF has been repeatedly shown to be down regulated both in HD patients as well as transgenic and knock-in HD mouse models. In this chapter we review the evidence implicating this important neurotrophic factor in the neuropathology of HD and discuss how increasing trophic support in the HD brain might be of potential clinical relevance for the treatment of this devastating neurodegenerative disorder.

Keywords: Brain-derived neurotrophic factor; Huntington's disease; transcription; transport; trophic support; therapy

Abbreviations

AdBDNF	adenoviral BDNF;
AdNoggin	adenoviral noggin;
BAC	bacterial artificial chromosome;
BDNF	brain-derived neurotrophic factor;
CAG	cytosine-adenine-guanine;
DARPP-32	dopamine- and cyclic-AMP-regulated phosphoprotein of molecular weight 32 kDa;
ELISA	enzyme-linked immunosorbent assay;
FDA	Food and Drug Administration;
GABA	gamma-aminobutyric acid;
HAP1	huntingtin-associated protein-1;
HD	Huntington's disease;
LTD	long-term depression;
LTP	long-term potentiation;
MAPK	mitogen-activated protein kinase;

NGF	nerve growth factor;
NF-κB	nuclear factor-κB;
NIIs	neuronal intranuclear inclusions;
NMDA	*N*-methyl-D-aspartate;
NRSF	Neuron-Restrictive Silencer Factor;
NT-3	neurotrophin-3;
NT-4	neurotrophin-4;
PI3K	phosphatidylinositol 3-kinase;
PKB/AKT	protein kinase B;
PKC	protein kinase C;
PLC γ	phospholipase C γ;
p75NTR	p75 neurotrophin receptor;
RE1	repressor element-1;
REST	RE1-Silencing Transcription factor;
SSRIs	selective serotonin re-uptake inhibitors;
Trk	tyrosine kinase receptor;
UHDRS	Unified Huntington's Disease Rating Scale;
YAC	yeast artificial chromosome

1. Huntington's Disease

Huntington's disease (HD) is a neurodegenerative disorder caused by an expansion in the number of cytosine-adenine-guanine (CAG) repeats in the *HD* gene. This gene is located on the short arm of chromosome 4 and encodes the protein huntingtin. Normally, the *HD* gene displays 6-36 CAG repeats, and HD develops if this number exceeds 37-39 (The Huntington's Disease Collaborative Research Group, 1993). The trinucleotide CAG encodes the amino acid glutamine. In HD, the increase in the number of CAG repeats results in a long stretch of polyglutamine residues that is located in the NH_2-terminal of the mutant protein and leads to its misfolding. It is now believed that mutant huntingtin acquires novel pathological functions as a consequence of this conformational change (for review see Gil and Rego, 2008; Zuccato et al., 2010).

Despite the fact that mutant huntingtin is ubiquitously expressed throughout life, in most cases the onset of HD symptoms does not occur until midlife, between the ages of 35 and 50 years. The disease progresses over time and is invariably fatal 15 to 20 years after the onset of the first symptoms, with the age of onset being negatively correlated to the number of CAG repeats

(Langbehn et al., 2010). Motor disturbances, associated with the loss of voluntary movement coordination and chorea, are the classical symptoms of HD with the appearance of subtle motor abnormalities during the pre-manifest stage being associated with a higher probability of disease onset and smaller striatal volumes (Biglan et al., 2009). Bradykinesia and rigidity appear in later stages of the disease, with juvenile forms (with CAG repeats over 60) often displaying tremor and epileptic seizures (for review see Gil and Rego, 2008). The majority of patients also suffer from severe weight loss and muscle wasting (Sanberg et al., 1981; Kirkwood et al., 2001; Djousse et al., 2002). Although the cause of these peripheral symptoms is still unclear, a number of endocrine abnormalities have also been reported to occur in patients with HD (for review see Petersen and Bjorkqvist, 2006), including increased levels of corticosteroids (Heuser et al., 1991; Leblhuber et al., 1995), reduced levels of testosterone (Markianos et al., 2005) and a high prevalence of diabetes mellitus (Podolsky et al., 1972; Farrer, 1985).

Longitudinal cognitive changes also occur in HD. Visuomotor integration deficits (characterized by deficits in speed, accuracy, and speed of error detection and correction) are evident many years before the clinical onset of HD (Say et al., 2011). During the early stages of the disease, cognitive impairment is not diffuse and homogeneous, but reflective of the relative sparing of higher cognitive functions (Caine et al., 1977). Verbal recall, verbal recognition and procedural memory may be impaired at this stage (Butters et al., 1985). Recently diagnosed patients may have retrograde amnesia with reduced remote memory (Albert et al., 1981). Performance in commonly used cognitive tests (such as the Symbol Digit, Circle Tracing, and Stroop word reading tests) significantly deteriorates during the early disease stages (Stout et al., 2012). Emotion recognition impairments exist across the HD spectrum, but aggravate as the disease progresses (Labuschagne et al., 2012). Other cognitive processes also become compromised, likely reflecting the early pathological involvement of the striatum (Huber and Paulson, 1987). Cognitive deficits become more extensive as the pathological involvement of the neocortex increases (Panegyres, 2004). Although the mechanisms underlying the sub-cortical dementia in HD are not fully understood, it is believed that pathological changes at multiple sites in the fronto-striatal circuitry are responsible for these cognitive deficits. Importantly, these can be predicted by specific reductions in the density of several markers of dopaminergic neurotransmission (such as D1 and D2 dopamine receptors, and the dopamine transporter) (Bäckman et al., 1997), as well as alterations in regional cerebral blood flow (Wolf et al., 2011) in these brain regions. The sub-cortical dementia is characterized by reduced speed of cognitive processing in the absence of deficits in memory acquisition and retrieval. Slowness of responses and an impairment of working memory without aphasia, apraxia or agnosia reflects the involvement of sub-cortical structures, in particular the basal ganglia and its frontal lobe connections (for review see Panegyres, 2004). The development of chorea appears to correlate with the severity of amnesia involving working memory, in accord with the pathological involvement of the basal ganglia and frontal lobes (Webb et al., 1987).

Neuropathologically, HD is characterized by the formation of ubiquitinated neuronal intranuclear inclusions (NIIs) that contain mutant huntingtin (DiFiglia et al., 1997). A progressive dysfunction and loss of neurons can be detected in the striatum and certain layers of the cerebral cortex. However, other brain regions can also be affected (for review see Vonsattel and DiFiglia, 1998), including the hypothalamus (Kremer et al., 1990, 1991; Kassubek et al., 2004; Petersen et al., 2005) and the hippocampus (Spargo et al., 1993; Rosas et al., 2003). Indeed, recent studies have shown structural changes in the cingulate cortex (Hobbs et al., 2011), sensorimotor cortex (Dumas et al., 2012), and hypothalamus (Soneson et al., 2010) in pre-manifest and prodormal HD, whereas disruption of motor, associative and limbic cortico-striatal circuits were shown to differentially contribute to the functional deficits observed during the early stages of the disease (Delmaire et al., 2012).

The genetic predictability of HD makes it potentially the most tractable of the neurodegenerative diseases for early intervention. The optimum time for the introduction of disease-modifying therapies is prior to the onset of symptoms (Tabrizi et al., 2011). Since the discovery of the HD gene in 1993 (The Huntington's Disease Collaborative Research Group, 1993), a number of new drug targets, drug discovery strategies, and therapeutic approaches have been devised (for review see Li et al., 2005; Gil and Rego, 2009; Gil-Mohapel, 2012; Brocardo and Gil-Mohapel, 2012, 2013). However, despite the efforts of a growing international HD research community, there is still no cure or satisfactory treatment for this neurodegenerative disease (for review see Brocardo and Gil-Mohapel, 2012, 2013). Indeed, commonly prescribed medications such as neuroleptics (used to alleviate some of the motor and psychiatric symptoms) may in fact aggravate other cognitive deficits associated with HD such as emotion recognition (Labuschagne et al., 2012).

This lack of effective treatments in turn lowers the impetus for individuals at risk to engage in genetic testing (Hayden, 2000). Given the devastating emotional costs of this disorder (Bombard et al., 2009, 2011), as well as the large financial burden these individuals impose upon society, understanding the neurodegenerative mechanisms that underlie neuronal loss in HD and developing a treatment regime for this neurodegenerative disorder are recognized priorities.

2. Brain-Derived Neurotrophic Factor (BDNF)

2.1. Neurotrophins

Neurotrophins are a family of polypeptide growth factors that are expressed both during development and throughout adulthood (Hofer et al., 1990; Yan et al., 1997). They play crucial roles both in the proper wiring of neural circuits and in the modulation of connections in the mature nervous system by influencing neuronal survival and differentiation as well as synapse formation and plasticity (Waterhouse and Xu, 2009). This family of molecules includes nerve growth factor (NGF), brain-derived neurotrophic factor (BDNF), as well as neurotrophin-3 (NT-3) and neurotrophin-4 (NT-4). Of these, BDNF is the best characterized in terms of its role in synaptic plasticity (Kossel et al., 2001; Levine et al., 1995, 1998; Lohof et al., 1993) and alterations in BDNF levels have been associated with many disease states, including schizophrenia, depression, Alzheimer's disease, Parkinson's disease, and HD (Diniz and Teixeira, 2011; Satomura et al., 2011; Teixeira et al., 2010).

BDNF is synthesized as a precursor protein known as pre-pro-BDNF that is cleaved into pro-BDNF, which can then be further cleaved into mature BDNF (Lessmann et al., 2003). Recent studies have suggested that pro-BDNF (35 kDa) is secreted in an activity-dependent manner along with the enzyme tissue plasminogen activator, which then cleaves pro-BDNF into mature BDNF (14 kDa) (Waterhouse and Xu, 2009). Interestingly, pro-BDNF and mature BDNF are known to activate different intracellular signaling pathways (Section 2.2; Woo et al., 2005; Matsumoto et al., 2008).

2.2. Neurotrophin Receptors and their Normal Functions

Each neurotrophin can signal through two different types of cell surface receptors — the tyrosine kinase receptor (Trk) and the p75 neurotrophin receptor (p75NTR). The extracellular domain of each of the Trk receptors consists of a cysteine-rich cluster followed by three leucine-rich repeats, another cysteine-rich cluster and two immunoglobulin-like domains. Each receptor spans the membrane once and is terminated with a cytoplasmic domain consisting of a tyrosine kinase surrounded by several tyrosines that serve as phosphorylation-dependent docking sites for cytoplasmic adaptors and enzymes. Ligand-induced receptor dimerization results in kinase activation; subsequent receptor autophosphorylation on multiple tyrosine residues creates specific binding sites for intracellular target proteins, which bind to the activated receptor via SH2 domains (Reichardt, 2006)

The three most common types of Trk receptors are TrkA, TrkB, and TrkC. The differences in the signaling pathways initiated by these distinct types of receptors are important for generating a diversity of biological responses. Each of these receptor types has different binding affinities to certain types of neurotrophins. NGF binds mostly to TrkA, mature BDNF and NT-4 to TrkB, and NT-3 to TrkC. In addition, NT-3 can activate the other Trk receptors with less efficiency (Barbacid, 1994; Reichardt, 2006).

In addition, all of the neurotrophins bind to the p75NTR, a member of the tumor necrosis receptor superfamily. The p75NTR contains an extracellular domain that includes four cysteine-rich motifs, a glycosylated extracellular region involved in ligand binding, a transmembrane region, and a short cytoplasmic sequence lacking intrinsic catalytic activity (Chao and Hempstead, 1995; Dechant and Barde, 2002). Neurotrophin binding to p75NTR is linked to several intracellular signal transduction pathways, including those mediated by nuclear factor-κB (NF-κB), Jun kinase and sphingo-myelin hydrolysis (Dechant and Barde, 2002). The p75NTR molecule serves as a pro-apoptotic receptor during developmental cell death and after injury to the nervous system (Roux and Barker, 2002). Moreover, cell death triggered by p75NTR signaling has been observed during conditions of stress, injury or inflammation (Dobrowsky and Carter, 2000; Lee et al., 2001). Furthermore, p75NTR modulates Trk receptor function in multiple ways, by promoting ligand binding and accessibility to neurotrophins through axon growth and target innervation, and by facilitating endocytosis and retrograde transport to membrane compartments where internal engagement of neurotrophins with Trk receptors may promote intracellular signaling

(Benedetti et al. 1993; Brennan et al. 1999; Curtis et al. 1995; Davies et al. 1993; Makkerh et al. 2005).

Importantly, while pro-BDNF signals through the low-affinity p75NTR that is believed to be involved in apoptosis (Lessmann et al., 2003; Roux and Barker, 2002; Teng et al., 2005), mature BDNF signals through the high-affinity TrkB receptor, stimulating cell survival by up-regulating the activity of survival genes and inhibiting the function of the proteins that lead to programmed cell death (Bhave et al., 1999; Encinas et al., 1999). Moreover, pro-BDNF and mature BDNF also appear to have opposite roles on synaptic plasticity, with pro-BDNF promoting long-term depression (LTD) and mature BDNF facilitating long-term potentiation (LTD) (Woo et al., 2005). Additionally, mature BDNF can also facilitate various synaptic reorganization processes, including formation and maintenance of dendrites and dendritic spines (McAllister et al., 1999).

When BDNF is bound to TrkB, it induces its dimerization and the receptor tyrosine kinase is autophosphorylated, leading to activation of intracellular signaling cascades, as well as augmentation of *N*-methyl-D-aspartate (NMDA) receptor currents (Levine et al., 1998). There are at least three signaling transduction pathways that BDNF-TrkB activation can regulate. The phospholipase C γ (PLC γ) pathway, which leads to activation of protein kinase C (PKC); the phosphatidylinositol 3-kinase (PI3K) pathway, which activates the serine/threonine protein kinase B (PKB/AKT); and the mitogen-activated protein kinase (MAPK) pathway, which activates several downstream effectors. Each of these signaling pathways confers the unique function of BDNF on cells (for review, see Mattson, 2008; Yoshii and Constantine-Paton, 2010). In brief, rapid synaptic and ion channel effects are thought to depend on PLC γ-mediated release of intracellular calcium stores, and longer-lasting effects involving transcription are considered to be downstream of PI3K and MAPK pathways. In addition, there is also evidence that BDNF may directly activate voltage-gated sodium channels to mediate rapid depolarization of target neurons (Blum et al., 2002).

3. Wild-Type *versus* Mutant Huntingtin and BDNF

Huntingtin is a ubiquitously expressed protein with a molecular mass of approximately 347 kDa and approximately 3,144 amino acids, depending on the number of glutamine residues present in its NH_2-terminal. Huntingtin is constitutively expressed throughout the body, being highly enriched in the brain (DiFiglia et al., 1995). Although it has been known since 1993 that an expansion in the number of glutamines in the NH_2-terminal of huntingtin is the underlying cause of HD (The Huntington's Disease Collaborative Research Group, 1993), the relevance of the polyglutamine tail to the actual function of the entire protein is not yet fully understood. However, this mutation is thought to confer a toxic gain of function as well as the loss of function of the normal protein (for review see Gil and Rego, 2008).

3.1. Regulation of BDNF Transcription by Huntingtin

The diversity of functions attributed to BDNF suggest that this important neurotrophin is subjected to sophisticated regulatory mechanisms, including tight and highly controlled mechanisms of gene expression, mRNA and protein transport, as well as regulated protein cleavage and processing (Greenberg et al., 2009). Wild type huntingtin is known to regulate transcription of multiple genes (for review see Gil and Rego, 2008), among which the gene encoding BDNF has received special attention (Zuccato et al., 2001, 2003). In an elegant study by Zuccato and collaborators (2003), wild type huntingtin was shown to interact with the transcriptional factor complex repressor-element-1 (RE1) transcription factor (REST) / neuron-restrictive silencer factor (NRSF) in the cytoplasm thus preventing this complex from translocating into the nucleus and binding to neuron-restrictive silencer element (NRSE) sequences and inhibiting gene transcription. Interestingly, the promoter of the *bdnf* gene contains an NRSE sequence, and therefore, in the presence of wild type huntingtin, this REST/NRSF-mediated mechanism of transcription inhibition is not favored and the transcription of the *bdnf* gene can occur (Zuccato et al., 2003). On the other hand, mutant huntingtin does not have the ability to bind and interact with NRSE-binding transcription factors (such as the REST/NRSF complex). In this case, the failure of mutant huntingtin to interact with REST/NRSF in the cytoplasm leads to its nuclear accumulation, where it binds to NRSE sequences and promotes histone deacetylation, leading to the remodeling of the chromatin into a closed structure. As a result, there is a suppression of NRSE-containing genes, including the *bdnf* gene (Zuccato et al., 2003). This is one case where the loss of the normal huntingtin function can have profound effects, leading to decreased levels of BDNF, an important survival factor for striatal neurons

(Altar et al., 1997; Baquet et al., 2004; Gauthier et al., 2004; Zuccato et al., 2001). Indeed, BDNF knock-out models were recently shown to largely recapitulate the expression profiling of human HD (Strand et al., 2007), suggesting that striatal medium-sized spiny neurons suffer similar insults in HD and BDNF-deprived environments (see Section 4.1).

3.2. Regulation of BDNF Transport by Huntingtin

Once transcription of the *bdnf* gene occurs, the large BDNF precursor protein (pre-pro-BDNF) is synthesized and subsequently processed by proteolytic cleavage and trafficked through the Golgi apparatus to the trans-Golgi network where it is packaged into secretory vesicles (Thomas and Davies, 2005). BDNF mRNA has been detected in many brain regions, including the cortex, hippocampus, amygdala, lateral hypothalamus, ventral tegmental area, substantia nigra and nucleus of the solitary tract (Conner et al., 1997; Xu et al., 2003). TrkB in the adult rat brain has been localized to the olfactory system, cortex, hippocampus, most nuclei of the hypothalamus, striatum, amygdala, septal nuclei, substantia nigra, cerebellar Purkinje cells, spinal motor neurons, and brainstem sensory nuclei (Masana et al., 1993; Kernie et al., 2000; Xu et al., 2003). However, not all areas that express TrkB are also sites of BDNF synthesis, though they may contain BDNF-positive fibers, a pattern seen in the striatum and arcuate hypothalamic nuclei (Altar et al., 1997; Xu et al., 2003; Baydyuk et al., 2011). Such brain areas are sites of anterograde or retrograde BDNF action, with BDNF originating from distal brain regions.

Indeed, the BDNF found in the striatum is synthesized and anterogradely transported from cell bodies located in the cerebral cortex, substantia nigra pars compacta, amygdala, and thalamus (Altar et al., 1997; Baquet et al., 2004). Since the striatum does not produce BDNF but depends on it for proper function, abnormalities in *bdnf* gene expression and anterograde transport of this neurotrophin in distal brain regions that supply BDNF to the striatum might contribute to striatal neuronal dysfunction and death as seen in HD (Gauthier et al., 2004; Zuccato et al., 2001).

Interestingly, as demonstrated by both *in vitro* and *in vivo* studies, wild type huntingtin is a positive regulatory factor for vesicular transport by interacting with vesicles and microtubules (Borrell-Pages et al., 2006) and facilitating vesicular transport in both anterograde and retrograde directions (Caviston et al., 2007; Gauthier et al., 2004; Gunawardena et al., 2003). This mechanism involves the direct interaction of wild type huntingtin with dynein intermediate chain (Caviston et al., 2007) and with huntingtin-associated protein-1 (HAP1), which in turn interacts with the p150Glued subunit of dynactin and kinesin (Engelender et al., 1997; Gauthier et al., 2004; McGuire et al., 2006). In an elegant study by Gauthier and colleagues (2004), wild type huntingtin was shown to promote neuronal survival by facilitating the transport of BDNF-containing vesicles along the microtubules. Consistent with the hypothesis of loss of wild type huntingtin function contributing to neurodegeneration in the HD brain (for review see Gil and Rego, 2008), a reduction in wild type huntingtin levels leads to attenuated BDNF trafficking. Indeed, an increase in the number of CAG repeats results in the abnormal association of mutant huntingtin with p150glued via HAP1, which in turn prevents the efficient movement of BDNF-containing vesicles along the microtubules. Furthermore, disruption of BDNF transport results not only in decreased neurotrophic support but also in increased neurotoxicity, which can then be rescued by wild type huntingtin (Gauthier et al., 2004). In agreement with this mechanism, Colin et al (2008) have also demonstrated that the function of huntingtin as a facilitator of neuronal anterograde and retrograde BDNF transport is regulated by the phosphorylation state of huntingtin at serine-421. Thus, when huntingtin is phosphorylated, kinesin-1 is recruited to vesicles and microtubules, facilitating anterograde transport of BDNF. In contrast, when huntingtin is not phosphorylated, kinesin-1 detaches and vesicles are more likely to undergo retrograde transport of BDNF. Importantly, this also applies to other vesicles, suggesting an essential role for huntingtin in the control of vesicular directionality in neurons (Colin et al., 2008).

In summary, both suppression of *bdnf* gene expression and deficient BDNF transport (mainly through the corticostriatal pathway), might concomitantly contribute to the reduced levels of BDNF that have been repeatedly shown in the striatum of both HD transgenic mouse models (see Section 4.1) and HD patients (see Section 4.2), thus providing strong evidence for a reduction in BDNF-mediated trophic support being a crucial factor in the pathogenesis of HD.

4. Evidence for Reduced Trophic Support in the HD Brain

4.1. Reduction in BDNF Expression in HD Genetic Mouse Models

Reduced BDNF protein and mRNA levels have been consistently reported in multiple genetic mouse models of HD. In particular, decreased BDNF protein levels have been found in the cortex, striatum and hippocampus of yeast artificial chromosome (YAC) 72 mice (Zuccato et al., 2001), which express full-length human huntingtin with 72 glutamines (Hodgson et al., 1999). Of note, a 30% reduction in cortical BDNF protein levels can be detected in these mice by 9 months of age (Zuccato et al., 2001), thus preceding the onset of the classical motor symptoms and striatal neuropathology characteristic of HD and suggesting that decreases in cortical trophic support may occur at an early stage during the course of the disease. On the other hand, the striatal reduction in BDNF protein content reported in this initial study (Zuccato et al., 2001), is in agreement with a subsequent study showing a decrease in BDNF mRNA levels in the striatum of YAC72 that could be detected as early as 3 months of age (Hermel et al., 2004). With regards to the hippocampus, the study by Zuccato et al. (2001) found a 40% reduction in BDNF protein content in this brain region.

Interestingly, while to date there are no studies on BDNF content in the hippocampus of a similar transgenic mouse model, the YAC128 mice (which express the full-length human *HD* gene with 128 CAG repeats; Slow et al., 2003), hippocampal-dependent cognitive deficits (Van Raamsdonk et al., 2005; Pouladi et al., 2009) and reductions in adult hippocampal neurogenesis (Simpson et al., 2011) have been reported to occur in this YAC model as early as 3 months of age, long before the onset of motor abnormalities and striatal neuropathology (Slow et al., 2003). As BDNF has been implicated in both hippocampal function (Lohof et al., 1993; Levine et al., 1995, 1998; Kossel et al., 2001; Woo et al., 2005) and adult neurogenesis (Zigova et al., 1998; Benraiss et al., 2001; Pencea et al., 2001), it is tempting to speculate that a reduction in hippocampal BDNF content may underlie, at least in part, alterations in hippocampal structural plasticity (Simpson et al., 2011) and hippocampal-dependent behaviours (Van Raamsdonk et al., 2005; Pouladi et al., 2009) seen in these mice. Future studies are thus warranted in order to test whether similar to what has been reported in YAC72 mice (Zuccato et al.,

2001), a reduction in hippocampal BDNF content is also observed in the YAC128 HD mouse model. Furthermore, these data may have a clinical correlation insofar as cognitive abnormalities can also be detected in pre-manifest HD carriers, years before the onset of the motor symptoms (Caine et al., 1977; Albert et al., 1981; Butters et al., 1985; Schmidtke et al., 2002; Stout et al., 2012; see Section 1).

In agreement with the findings from the YAC72 mouse model, Gray and colleagues (2008) also found a decrease in BDNF transcription in the brains of a different full-length transgenic mouse model, the bacterial artificial chromosome (BAC) HD transgenic mice (which express full-length mutant huntingtin with 103 CAG repeats under endogenous huntingtin regulation). Interestingly, in this model the decrease in BDNF parallels the onset of locomotor deficits (Gray et al., 2008). Whether these two events are related is an interesting hypothesis that deserves further investigation.

Similarly to the findings obtained with the full-length models, several studies have also found alterations in BDNF levels in the brains of various truncated models of HD, which express different NH_2-terminal portions of the mutant protein. In R6/2 mice, which express an NH_2-terminal fragment of mutant huntigtin bearing approximately 145 glutamine residues corresponding to about 3% of the entire protein (Mangiarini et al., 1996), a 50% reduction in BDNF protein levels was observed in the brain at 12 weeks of age (Zhang et al., 2003) (i.e., when animals are symptomatic and show motor abnormalities and striatal neuropathology; Mangiarini et al., 1996). At this age, a 20% reduction in perikarial BDNF mRNA was also detected in layer V cortical neurons (which project to the striatum) (Wang et al., 2006) and subsequent studies have indicated that a decrease in BDNF mRNA can be observed in the cortex of these HD mice as early as 4-5 weeks of age, when animals are still in the pre-symptomatic stage (Zuccato et al., 2005). Furthermore, a reduction in *bdnf* gene transcription was also shown to occur in the cerebellum of 8 weeks old R6/2 mice (Luthi-Carter et al., 2002). Whether this reduction in trophic support in the cerebellum results in cerebellar dysfunction (which in turn can contribute to the motor coordination deficits observed in these mice and human HD patients) is an interesting possibility that deserves future investigations.

More recently, Peng and collaborators (2008) have shown that significant reductions in the protein levels of BDNF can also be detected in the hippocampus of 10 week-old R6/2 mice (Peng et al., 2008). Of note, various studies have found significant reductions in adult hippocampal neurogenesis (Gil et al., 2004, 2005), synaptic plasticity (Murphy et al., 2000), and hippocampal-dependent learning and memory (Murphy et al. 2000) in these transgenic HD mice. Importantly, these hippocampal abnormalities can be detected early on during the course of the disease and before animals start showing an overt motor phenotype. Again, since BDNF has been linked with both structural (Zigova et al., 1998; Benraiss et al., 2001; Pencea et al., 2001) and functional (Lohof et al., 1993; Levine et al., 1995, 1998; Kossel et al., 2001; Woo et al., 2005) plasticity, it will be interesting to determine whether reduced hippocampal BDNF levels underlie the development of these hippocampal deficits in R6/2 mice.

Interestingly, the reductions in BDNF levels that are seen in the R6/2 brain are also accompanied by a progressive decrease in the levels of BDNF mRNA in peripheral blood. These results indicate that blood BDNF mRNA levels may be used as an accessible biomarker to assess disease progression and drug efficacy in HD rodent models (Conforti et al., 2008).

Brain BDNF levels have also been evaluated with conflicting results in the R6/1 line, which expresses a similar N-terminal fragment of mutant huntingtin to that used to generate the R6/2 line but bearing approximately 115 glutamine residues. As a consequence, R6/1 mice show a slower disease progression than their R6/2 counterparts (Mangiarini et al., 1996). Thus, while Spires et al. (2004) reported that BDNF protein levels were reduced in the R6/1 striatum but not in the cerebral cortex at 5 months of age, Canals et al. (2004) found no deficiency in striatal BDNF protein levels at the age of 6 months. On the other hand, Pang et al. (2006) have found unchanged BDNF protein levels in the striatum and hippocampus of 5-month-old R6/1 mice, while increased levels were detected in the frontal cortex. Furthermore, despite no deficits in cortical, striatal and hippocampal protein levels, these authors reported a decrease in BDNF mRNA levels in these brain regions (Pang et al., 2006). The discrepancies between studies may be due, at least in part, to differences in the methods used for BDNF protein quantification. Indeed, while the study by Spires et al. (2004) used Western-blotting, which differentiates between mature BDNF (which decreased) from pro-BDNF (which remained unchanged), the studies by Canals et al. (2004) and Pang et al. (2006) used a BDNF enzyme-linked immunosorbent assay (ELISA), which despite being more quantitative does not differentiate between the mature and immature forms of BDNF. Thus, it is possible that in these HD mice the levels of mature BDNF are significantly decreased but the levels of the much more abundant immature BDNF (i.e., pro-BDNF) remain largely unchanged (Pang et al., 2006). If this is the case, these results may suggest a disruption of intracellular BDNF processing. Thus, even though total levels of BDNF (i.e., pro-BDNF plus mature BDNF) are unaltered, there might be a shift in the normal balance between pro-BDNF and mature BDNF towards an increase in pro-BDNF. As mature BDNF and pro-BDNF are though to have opposite roles in signal transduction, with pro-BDNF acting as a pro-apoptotic signaling molecule and mature BDNF as a pro-survival activator (see Section 2.2), this imbalance in the ratio between mature BDNF and pro-BDNF might result in an increased activation of pro-apoptotic intracellular cascades, which ultimately will result in neuronal degeneration. Furthermore, deficits in total *bdnf* gene expression and alterations in the levels of the various *bdnf* gene transcripts have been noted in the hippocampus of 12 weeks-old R6/1 mice (Zajac et al., 2010). Of note and similarly to the findings in the R6/2 transgenic line (Gil et al., 2004, 2005), deficits in adult hippocampal neurogenesis have also been found in R6/1 mice (Lazic et al., 2004, 2006), further indicating that a reduction in *bdnf* gene expression and/or BDNF protein levels may underlie the reduced neurogenic capacity that has been repeatedly reported in transgenic mouse models of HD.

In agreement with the evidence from the R6 lines, Duan and colleagues (2003) have also found a 70-80% reduction in striatal and cortical protein BDNF levels in 3 month-old N171-82Q HD transgenic mice (which express a cDNA encoding an NH_2-terminal fragment of huntingtin with 171 amino acids bearing 82 glutamines; Schilling et al., 1999). Furthermore, significant reductions in striatal and cortical BDNF protein levels have also been found in 5 month-old homozygous HD knock-in mice (engineered by introduction of 111 CAG repeats into the mouse *Hdh* gene) (Gines et al., 2003). Additional results from Borrell-Pages et al. (2006) showing that at 3 months of age these homozygous knock-in HD mice already present a non-significant trend towards a reduction in BDNF protein levels in the brain suggest that the decrease in trophic support observed in older animals (Gines et al., 2003) might indeed initiate earlier in the course of the disease. Moreover, a study by Simmons et al. (2009) also found that BDNF protein levels were reduced by 40–45% in the hippocampus, cortex and striatum of 2-month old homozygous knock-in mice, further supporting the idea that reductions in BDNF occur early on in the brains of knock-in HD mice (Simmons et al., 2009).

Finally, a very interesting study by Strand and colleagues (2007) has demonstrated that the pattern of striatal gene expression found in both heterozygous and homozygous *bdnf* knock-out mice resembles human HD (even more so than other commonly used HD rodent models such as the R6/2 mice) (Strand et al., 2007), further implicating a reduction in trophic support in striatal degeneration in the HD brain.

4.2. Reduction in BDNF Expression in the Human HD Brain

To date, a few studies have also analyzed whether BDNF levels are altered in the human HD brain (Ferrer et al., 2000; Zuccato et al., 2001; Gauthier et al., 2004).

In the first study the parietal cortex, temporal cortex, hippocampus, caudate and putamen of four grade III HD subjects were analyzed and compared with samples from six age-matched controls and a significant decrease in BDNF levels was observed in the HD striatum but not in the other brain regions analyzed (Ferrer et al., 2000). Specifically, the levels of mature BDNF were shown to be reduced by 53% in the caudate and by 82% in the putamen of the HD subjects, while being unchanged in the cerebral (parietal and temporal) cortex and the hippocampus. As no differences in BDNF cortical levels were detected in this study, the authors suggested that the reduction in striatal BDNF protein levels was the result of selective defects in striatal neurons themselves rather than reduced BDNF input from the cerebral cortex (Ferrer et al., 2000). These results were supported by the findings of Gauthier et al. (2004), showing that BDNF protein levels were reduced to about 50% in striatum, but not the cerebral cortex, of 10 HD patients as compared to 7 controls (Gauthier et al., 2004).

However, a study by Zuccato et al. (2001) found a 50% reduction in the levels of total BDNF (as assessed by ELISA) and BDNF mRNA in the frontoparietal cortex of two HD subjects (grade II) in comparison with two age-matched controls (Zuccato et al., 2001). Differences in the methods used to determine BDNF levels (i.e., evaluation of pro-BDNF and mature BDNF levels by western-blotting versus assessment of total BDNF levels by ELISA) and in the samples analyzed (different stages of disease progression, numbers of CAG repeats, and age of the patients at the time of death) may have largely contributed to these discrepant results. Nevertheless, it is clear from these studies that BDNF is indeed reduced in the human HD striatum.

In an attempt to determine whether similar decreases in BDNF levels could be detected in serum samples from HD patients, Ciammola and colleagues (2007) compared BDNF serum levels between 42 HD patients and 42 age-matched healthy subjects. Interestingly, serum BDNF levels were shown to be significantly lower in HD patients than in age-matched healthy controls. Furthermore, lower BDNF levels were associated with longer CAG repeat lengths and longer duration of illness. On the other hand, severity of the illness, as assessed by the Unified Huntington's Disease Rating Scale (UHDRS) motor and cognitive scores, was negatively related to serum BDNF levels (Ciammola et al., 2007). Although promising, the results from this initial work were not replicated in a more recent study that evaluated BDNF levels in 398 blood samples including 138 controls, 56 pre-manifest HD individuals, and 204 HD patients (Zuccato et al., 2011). In this study, no significant differences in either plasma or serum BDNF protein levels were seen between groups. Furthermore, no differences in BDNF mRNA levels in blood samples from 47 controls, 25 pre-manifest HD individuals, and 70 HD patients were found (Zuccato et al., 2011). Thus, despite the well-established reductions in brain levels of this neurotrophic factor, its measurement in human blood does not appear to be a reliable biomarker candidate to monitor HD progression in the human population.

5. Increasing Trophic Support as a Therapeutic Intervention for HD

5.1. Direct Up-Regulation of Striatal BDNF Levels

Various studies have assessed the effects of up-regulating BDNF protein levels or gene expression in different animal models of HD. In most cases, delivery of BDNF by protein infusion through the implantation of BDNF mini-pumps (Canals et al., 2004), intrastriatal injection of adenovirus expressing *bdnf* (Cho et al., 2007; Kells et al., 2004), or implantation of cells expressing *bdnf* (Frim et al., 1993, Martinez-Serrano and Bjorklund, 1996; Perez-Navarro et al., 1999, 2000; Ryu et al., 2004) were shown to induce some degree of striatal neuroprotection and motor improvement (for review see Sari, 2011; Zuccato and Cattaneo, 2007; Zuccato et al., 2010).

For example, the delivery of BDNF into the striatum of R6/1 mice using osmotic mini-pumps was shown to reduce the degeneration of gamma-aminobutryic acid (GABA)ergic/enkephalinergic striatal projection neurons, which is the most affected neuronal population in the HD brain. Furthermore, BDNF infusions also delayed motor impairments and improved the survival of R6/1 mice (Canals et al., 2004). Despite these promising results, the use of mini-pumps presents with some disadvantages that should be taken into consideration when extrapolating these results to the clinic. First, the degree of invasiveness of this procedure might not be practical or even feasible in the clinical setting. Second, this administration route will likely generate a steep concentration gradient, originating from the infusion point, which could lead to alterations in the infused tissue and the development of adverse side effects, such as edema (Gill et al., 2003). Thus, other approaches to efficiently deliver optimum doses of BDNF to the brain are currently considered more feasible candidates for clinical trials in HD.

An attractive alternative approach is gene therapy using viral vectors containing the *bdnf* gene, which allows for the constant and local production of the protein by the desired neuronal population. Moreover, gene therapy also overcomes the problem of protein instability that may result from the long-term storage of BDNF inside the pumps. Given this rationale, Cho and colleagues (2007) have tested the potential beneficial effects of administering a combination of adenoviral BDNF (AdBDNF) and adenoviral noggin (AdNoggin) via intraventricular injections to 4- and 6-week old R6/2 mice. A combination of both AdBDNF and AdNoggin was shown to increase the recruitment of new neurons from the subventricular zone into the striatum of R6/2 mice. Furthermore, these newly generated neurons were shown to mature into dopamine- and cyclic-AMP-regulated phosphoprotein of molecular weight 32 kDa (DARPP-32)-positive GABA-ergic medium-sized spiny neurons that expressed either enkephalin or substance P and extended fibers to the globus pallidus. Importantly, AdBDNF/AdNoggin treatment also improved rotarod performance and open-field activity and increased the survival of R6/2 mice by 16.8% (Cho et al., 2007). Nevertheless and although *bdnf* gene therapy appears as a promising candidate for clinical trials, there are still a few drawbacks that should be overcome before this strategy can be used in the clinical setting. The first problem is the regulation of the amount of BDNF produced locally, as an excess of total BDNF can potentially be deleterious, namely if the mechanisms of BDNF processing are compromised, leading to the accumulation of increased amounts of pro-BDNF, which, as stated above (see Section 2.2), is known to have pro-apoptotic functions (Teng et al., 2005). Secondly, transduction is often associated with inflammation, which may also result from vector toxicity and prevent long-term therapy. Another major problem is the risk of accidental insertional mutagenesis by viral vectors and subsequent tumor formation (Hacein-Bey-Abina et al., 2008). To overcome these problems, new adeno-associated viral vectors lacking pathogenicity and immunogenicity as well as nontoxic viral systems are currently being investigated (Biffi and Naldini, 2005; Yanez-Munoz et al., 2006).

Another alternative to increasing BDNF levels locally is by striatal transplantation of cells engineered to stably express BDNF. This approach has been tested in animal models of HD, using either immortalized rat fibroblasts genetically engineered to secrete BDNF, or human embryonic neural progenitors (Frim et al., 1993, Martinez-Serrano and Bjorklund, 1996; Perez-Navarro et al., 1999, 2000; Ryu et al., 2004). Overall, these strategies resulted in improved motor performance and reduced striatal neuropathology (for review see Zuccato and Cattaneo, 2007). Since xenogenic grafts can be rejected by the host and immortalized cells can cause tumor growth, research is currently focused on the development of stable, non-tumorigenic human neural stem cell lines that can express BDNF (for review see Conti and Cattaneo, 2010; Rossi and Cattaneo, 2002).

5.2. Up-Regulation of BDNF Levels by Pharmacological Strategies

Several studies have tested the ability of different pharmacological interventions in increasing endogenous BDNF levels using *in vivo* models of HD. These strategies would circumvent the problems related with the use of invasive methods of BDNF delivery while allowing for the correct dosage and stability of this neurotrophin.

Within this scenario, the noncompetitive inhibitor of ionotropic glutamate NMDA receptors riluzole has been shown to increase BDNF expression (Squitieri et al., 2009) and ameliorate HD symptoms in both HD transgenic mouse models (Schiefer et al., 2002; Hockly et al., 2006) and human HD patients (Squitieri et al., 2009). On the other hand, cystamine, an inhibitor of transglutaminase, is a neuroprotective drug that inhibits caspase-3 activation (Lesort et al., 2003) and increases the levels of the antioxidants glutathione and L-cysteine (Fox et al., 2004; Lesort et al., 2003). Furthermore, cystamine has been shown to increase the transport and release of BDNF from brain neurons (Borrell-Pages, 2006). In agreement, cystamine and its Food and Drug Administration (FDA)-approved derivative cysteamine were shown to be effective in increasing BDNF levels and consequently inducing neuroprotective effects in HD mouse models and in up-regulating serum BDNF levels in mouse and primate models of HD (Borrell-Pages et al., 2006).

BDNF can also be regulated by activation of the serotonergic system (for review see Powrozek et al., 2004), and administration of selective serotonin re-uptake inhibitors (SSRIs) was shown to increase the levels of BDNF in the hippocampus (Gewirtz et al., 2002; Vaidya et al., 1997, 1999; for review see Duman, 1998). Thus, SSRIs might be used to modulate the levels of BDNF in the HD brain. In agreement, various studies have shown that treatment with different SSRIs can have beneficial effects on disease progression in HD transgenic models. Paroxetine was found to attenuate motor dysfunction and body weight loss, while increasing the life span of HD N171-82Q mice (Duan et al., 2004). Fluoxetine treatment rescued the deficits in hippocampal neurogenesis and improved hippocampal-dependent cognitive function in R6/1 mice, although no effects on the locomotor deficits and the loss of body weight were observed (Grote et al., 2005). In a more recent study, daily administration of sertraline to R6/2 mice (starting at 6 weeks of age) had no effect on the loss of body weight or the number of NIIs. However, sertraline-treated mice survived longer, performed better on the rotarod test and showed reduced striatal atrophy. Importantly, sertraline also ameliorated the impairment in hippocampal neurogenesis and attenuated the depletion of BDNF in the striatum and hippocampus of these HD mice (Peng et al., 2008). Similar results were also found in the N171-82Q HD transgenic mouse model (Duan et al., 2008). Indeed, although not affecting body weight or the number of NIIs in these mice, sertraline treatment was shown to improve their brain atrophy, motor performance, and survival (Duan et al., 2008). Furthermore, sertraline-treated N171-82Q HD mice also had normalized cortical BDNF and striatal serotonin levels as well as enhanced adult neurogenesis, which might mediate, at least in part, the beneficial effects of sertraline in these mice (Duan et al., 2008). Importantly, the serum and brain levels of sertraline that were shown to be beneficial in these transgenic mice are comparable to the levels achieved in humans treated with this antidepressant (Slaughter et al., 2001), making sertraline an interesting candidate for HD clinical trials.

5.3. Up-Regulation of BDNF Levels by Non-Invasive Strategies

Alternative approaches to increase BDNF levels in the brain include the use of environmental enrichment (Young et al., 1999; Ickes et al., 2000), physical exercise (Neeper et al., 1995, 1996; Oliff et al., 1998), and/or dietary restriction (Duan et al., 2001a, 2001b; Lee et al., 2000, 2002). Importantly, these are less-invasive and more cost effective strategies that are associated with very limited side effects.

Environmental stimulation has been linked with increased synaptic signaling and spine density (for review see Olson et al., 2006; Gil-Mohapel et al., 2010), up-regulation of adult neurogenesis (Kempermann et al., 1997), as well as increased levels of neurotrophins including BDNF (Young et al., 1999; Ickes et al., 2000). Usually, enriched conditions involve complex inanimate and social stimulation that allow for increased learning opportunities and exploration, increased social interaction, and more physical activity. Importantly, environmental enrichment has been repeatedly shown to delay the onset and progression of HD in transgenic mice (Carter et al., 2000; van Dellen et al., 2000; Hockly et al., 2002; Schilling et al., 2004; Spires et al., 2004; Lazic et al., 2006; reviewed in Gil and Rego, 2009; Gil-Mohapel et al., 2010). The initial study by van Dellen and colleagues (2000) demonstrated that exposure of R6/1 mice to an enriched environment delayed the onset of motor symptoms, decreased the severity of the clasping phenotype, and reduced the loss of peristriatal cerebral volume. Subsequent studies demonstrated that environmental enrichment could also slow disease progression in R6/2 (Hockly et al., 2002) and N171-82Q (Schilling et al., 2004) transgenic HD mice. Furthermore, environmental enrichments was shown to ameliorate the deficits in hippocampal neurogenesis observed in R6/1 mice (Lazic et al., 2006). In addition, environmental stimulation has been shown to delay the onset of cognitive deficits in this transgenic HD mouse model. Indeed, both short-term hippocampal-dependent memory and long-term spatial memory were both improved in R6/1 mice housed in enriched conditions (Nithianantharajah et al., 2009). Moreover, the beneficial effects of environmental stimulation have also been demonstrated in HD patients, where a more stimulating environment was shown to improve physical, mental and social functioning, even in late-stage HD affected individuals (Sullivan et al., 2001).

Whether the effects of environmental enrichment on neurogenic and cognitive functions were mediated by BDNF is an interesting possibility. In agreement with this hypothesis, studies in R6/1 mice have shown that environmental enrichment rescues hippocampal and striatal BDNF protein deficits, the latter by possibly promoting the anterograde transport of this neurotrophin from the anterior cortex to the striatum (Spires et al., 2004). However, a recent study by the same group subsequently found that environmental enrichment was unable to increase hippocampal BDNF mRNA levels in this transgenic HD mouse model (Zajac et al., 2010). Nevertheless, an increase in hippocampal BDNF protein levels may mediate, at least in part, the beneficial effects of environmental enrichment on adult hippocampal neurogenesis as well as learning and memory. Importantly, the beneficial effects of environmental stimulation have also been demonstrated in HD patients, where a more stimulating environment was shown to improve physical, mental and social functioning, even in late-stage HD affected individuals (Sullivan et al., 2001).

Physical activity is another non-invasive strategy known to stimulate adult hippocampal neurogenesis (van Praag et al., 1999a, 199b) and cognitive function (for review see Pang and Hannan, 2013), and to increase BDNF levels (Neeper et al., 1995, 1996; Oliff et al., 1998). In line with this evidence, various studies have now investigated the effects of physical exercise in transgenic mouse models of HD. Although a 4-week running period failed to increase hippocampal neurogenesis in R6/2 mice (Kohl et al., 2007), it might be that in this study HD mice simply did not exercise enough due to their severe locomotor impairments (Mangiarini et al., 1996). In fact, other studies that examined the effects of physical exercise on disease progression found that this non-invasive strategy was able to delay the onset of rear-paw clasping and ameliorate cognitive deficits in R6/1 mice when initiated in adulthood (Pang et al., 2006), and to delay the onset of deficits in motor coordination when initiated at a juvenile age (van Dellen et al., 2008). Unfortunately, physical exercise had no effect on the neuropathology of these mice since the shrinkage of the striatum and the anterior cingulate cortex, the overall decrease in brain weight, and the density of striatal ubiquitinated protein aggregates were not affected by exercise (Pang et al., 2006; van Dellen et al., 2008). Whether the beneficial effects of physical exercise on motor (Pang et al., 2006; van Dellen et al., 2008) and cognitive (Pang et al., 2006) deficits were mediated by an increase in BDNF levels is still under debate. Indeed, while Pang and collaborators (2006) reported that striatal and hippocampal BDNF protein levels remained unchanged in R6/1 transgenic mice that had free access to a running wheel (Pang et al., 2006), a more recent study found that wheel-running significantly increased total BDNF gene expression specifically in R6/1 female mice whereas no differences were detected in R6/1 males (Zajac et al., 2010). Differences in running distances between males and females might account for this sex-specific discrepancies in BDNF levels. Furthermore, as discussed above (see Section 4.1) differences in the methods used to evaluate BDNF levels may also contribute to the discrepant results obtain in these studies.

Finally, an elegant study by Duan et al. (2003) has shown that an intermittent fasting dietary restriction regimen, in which HD N171-82Q transgenic mice were deprived of food for a 24-hour period every other day, normalizes brain glucose metabolism and BDNF levels, delays the onset and slows the progression of the motor dysfunction, and increases the survival of these mice (Duan et al., 2003). These results suggest that the protective effects of dietary restriction may be mediated through an increase in BDNF levels and indicate that caloric restriction might be a feasible life-style change for patients with HD.

5.4. Future Directions

Since the mechanisms of reduced BDNF gene transcription (Section 3.1) and protein transport (Section 3.2) in the HD brain have been elucidated, a valid option to restore trophic support in the HD brain could be to pharmacologically target these specific mechanisms known to be responsible for BDNF dysfunction. For example, BDNF vesicle transport is known to depend on huntingtin phosphorylation at serine-421 (Colin et al., 2008). In agreement, Pineda et al. (2009) found that pharmacological inhibition of calcineurin (an huntingtin serine-421 phosphatase), restored BDNF transport defects observed in HD. On the other hand, identification of pharmacological compounds that could alleviate the REST/NRSF-dependent repression and consequently ameliorate the global transcription repression (and decreased BDNF-mediated trophic support) in the diseased brain (Rigamonti et al., 2007) might prove to be beneficial in HD. These strategies, which act specifically on well-defined molecular dysfunctions that underlie the reductions in BDNF levels in the HD brain, could be more effective in restoring trophic support and improve the development and progression of the disease than drugs that increase BDNF levels but do not specifically target a disease mechanism.

Conclusion

HD is a multifactorial neurodegenerative disorder, characterized by a variety of symptoms that range from severe motor deficits to profound cognitive dysfunction. Although the exact mechanisms of neurodegeneration that occur in the HD brain are still under investigation, several lines of evidence suggest that a decrease in trophic support (and in particular in the levels of BDNF) might underlie not only the demise of striatal neurons but also of neuronal populations in other brain regions, including the cortex and the hippocampus. Indeed, a reduction in BDNF levels might render striatal neurons more susceptible to the deleterious effects of mutant huntingtin and increase their susceptibility towards glutamate-mediated excitotoxicity and cell death. On the other hand, a decrease in hippocampal levels of this neurotrophin might underlie the deficits in hippocampal structural and functional (i.e., synaptic) plasticity that have been repeatedly reported to occur in various HD transgenic mouse models and contribute to some of the cognitive deficits observed in HD afflicted individuals.

As such, strategies aimed at restoring and increasing trophic support to these critical brain regions are likely to have a beneficial impact in slowing the progression and mitigating some of the symptoms associated with this devastating neurodegenerative disorder. Future studies are thus warranted in order to further develop safe and well-tolerated genetic or pharmacological strategies to increase the levels of neurotrophins such as BDNF in a clinically relevant way. Furthermore, life-style modifications that include an enriched environment (with multiple sources and types of stimulations), physical exercise, and caloric restriction might be additionally beneficial in potentiating the endogenous production of BDNF and its utilization by the target tissues in the brain. The implementation of such non-invasive therapeutic strategies as part of standard care should therefore be strongly encouraged.

Acknowledgments

P.S.B. and J.G.M. acknowledge funding from the *Ciência Sem Fronteiras* funding program (Science Without Borders, Brazilian Federal Government, Brazil).

References

Albert MS, Butters N, Brandt J. (1981) Development of remote memory loss in patients with Huntington's disease. *J. Clin. Neuropsychol.* 3: 1-12.

Altar CA, Cai N, Bliven T, Juhasz M, Conner JM, Acheson AL, Lindsay RM, Wiegand SJ. (1997) Anterograde transport of brain-derived neurotrophic factor and its role in the brain. *Nature* 389: 856-860.

Bäckman L, Robins-Wahlin TB, Lundin A, Ginovart N, Farde L. (1997) Cognitive deficits in Huntington's disease are predicted by dopaminergic *Brain* 120: 2207-2217.

Baquet ZC, Gorski JA, Jones KR (2004) Early striatal dendrite deficits followed by neuron loss with advanced age in the absence of anterograde cortical brain-derived neurotrophic factor. *J. Neurosci*. 24: 4250-4258.

Barbacid M (1994) The Trk family of neurotrophin receptors. *J. Neurobiol.* 25: 1386-1403.

Baydyuk M, Nguyen MT, Xu B (2011) Chronic deprivation of TrkB signaling leads to selective late-onset nigrostriatal dopaminergic degeneration. *Exp. Neurol.* 228: 118-125.

Benedetti M, Levi A, Chao MV (1993) Differential expression of nerve growth factor receptors leads to altered binding affinity and neurotrophin responsiveness. *Proc. Natl. Acad. Sci. U S A* 90: 7859-7863.

Benraiss A, Chmielnicki E, Lerner K, Roh D, Goldman SA. (2001) Adenoviral brain-derived neurotrophic factor induces both neostriatal and olfactory neuronal recruitment from endogenous progenitor cells in the adult forebrain. *J. Neurosci.* 21: 6718-6731.

Bhave SV, Ghoda L, Hoffman PL (1999) Brain-derived neurotrophic factor mediates the anti-apoptotic effect of NMDA in cerebellar granule neurons: signal transduction cascades and site of ethanol action. *J. Neurosci.* 19: 3277-3286.

Biffi A, Naldini L. (2005) Gene therapy of storage disorders by retroviral and lentiviral vectors. *Hum. Gene. Ther.* 16: 1133–1142.

Biglan KM, Ross CA, Langbehn DR, Aylward EH, Stout JC, Queller S, Carlozzi NE, Duff K, Beglinger LJ, Paulsen JS; PREDICT-HD Investigators of the Huntington Study Group. (2009) Motor abnormalities in premanifest persons with Huntington's disease: the PREDICT-HD study. *Mov. Disord.* 24: 1763-1772.

Blum R, Kafitz KW, Konnerth A (2002) Neurotrophin-evoked depolarization requires the sodium channel Na(V)1.9. *Nature* 419: 687-693.

Bombard Y, Palin J, Friedman JM, Veenstra G, Creighton S, Paulsen JS, Bottorff JL, Hayden MR; Canadian Respond-HD Collaborative Research Group. (2011) Factors associated with experiences of genetic discrimination among individuals at risk for Huntington disease. *Am. J. Med. Genet. B. Neuropsychiatr. Genet.* 156B: 19-27.

Bombard Y, Veenstra G, Friedman JM, Creighton S, Currie L, Paulsen JS, Bottorff JL, Hayden MR; Canadian Respond-HD Collaborative Research Group. (2009) Perceptions of genetic discrimination among people at risk for Huntington's disease: a cross sectional survey. *BMJ* 338: b2175.

Borrell-Pages M, Canals JM, Cordelieres FP, Parker JA, Pineda JR, Grange G, Bryson EA, Guillermier M, Hirsch E, Hantraye P, Cheetham ME, Neri C, Alberch J, Brouillet E, Saudou F, Humbert S. (2006) Cystamine and cysteamine increase brain levels of BDNF in Huntington disease via HSJ1b and transglutaminase. *J. Clin. Invest.* 116: 1410–1424.

Borrell-Pages M, Zala D, Humbert S, Saudou F (2006) Huntington's disease: from huntingtin function and dysfunction to therapeutic strategies. *Cell Mol. Life Sci.* 63: 2642-2660.

Brennan C, Rivas-Plata K, Landis SC (1999) The p75 neurotrophin receptor influences NT-3 responsiveness of sympathetic neurons in vivo. *Nat. Neurosci.* 2: 699-705.

Brocardo PS, Gil-Mohapel JM. (2012) Therapeutic strategies for Huntington's disease: from the bench to the clinic. *Current Psychopharmacology* 1: 137-154.

Brocardo PS, Gil-Mohapel JM. (2013) From preclinical to clinical trials: an update on potential therapies for Huntington's disease. *Current Psychopharmacology* 2: (in press).

Butters N, Wolfe J, Martone M, Granholm E, Cermak LS. (1985) Memory disorders associated with Huntington's disease: verbal recall, verbal recognition and procedural memory. *Neuropsychologia* 23: 729-743.

Caine ED, Ebert MH, Weingartner H. (1977) An outline for the analysis of dementia. The memory disorder of Huntington's disease. *Neurology* 27: 1087–1092.

Canals JM, Pineda JR, Torres-Peraza JF, Bosch M, Martín-Ibañez R, Muñoz MT, Mengod G, Ernfors P, Alberch J. (2004) Brain-derived neurotrophic factor regulates the onset and severity of motor dysfunction associated with enkephalinergic neuronal degeneration in Huntington's disease. *J. Neurosci.* 24: 7727-7739.

Carter RJ, Hunt MJ, Morton AJ. (2000) Environmental stimulation increases survival in mice transgenic for exon 1 of the Huntington's disease gene. *Mov. Disord.* 15: 925-937.

Caviston JP, Ross JL, Antony SM, Tokito M, Holzbaur EL (2007) Huntingtin facilitates dynein/dynactin-mediated vesicle transport. *Proc. Natl. Acad. Sci. U S A* 104: 10045-10050.

Chao MV, Hempstead BL (1995) p75 and Trk: a two-receptor system. *Trends Neurosci.* 18: 321-326.

Chen ZY, Ieraci A, Teng H, Dall H, Meng CX, Herrera DG, Nykjaer A, Hempstead BL, Lee FS. (2005) Sortilin controls intracellular sorting of brain-derived neurotrophic factor to the regulated secretory pathway. *J. Neurosci.* 25: 6156-6166.

Cho SR, Benraiss A, Chmielnicki E, Samdani A, Economides A, Goldman SA. (2007) Induction of neostriatal neurogenesis slows disease progression in a transgenic murine model of Huntington disease. *J. Clin. Invest.* 117: 2889–2902.

Ciammola A, Sassone J, Cannella M, Calza S, Poletti B, Frati L, Squitieri F, Silani V. (2007) Low brain-derived neurotrophic factor (BDNF) levels in serum of Huntington's disease patients. *Am. J. Med. Genet.* B *Neuropsychiatr. Genet.* 144B: 574-577.

Colin E, Zala D, Liot G, Rangone H, Borrell-Pages M, Li XJ, Saudou F, Humbert S. (2008) Huntingtin phosphorylation acts as a molecular switch for anterograde/retrograde transport in neurons. *EMBO J.* 27: 2124-2134.

Conforti P, Ramos C, Apostol BL, Simmons DA, Nguyen HP, Riess O, Thompson LM, Zuccato C, Cattaneo E. (2008) Blood level of brain-derived neurotrophic factor mRNA is progressively reduced in rodent models of Huntington's disease: restoration by the neuroprotective compound CEP-1347. *Mol. Cell Neurosci.* 39(1):1-7.

Conner JM, Lauterborn JC, Yan Q, Gall CM, Varon S (1997) Distribution of brain-derived neurotrophic factor (BDNF) protein and mRNA in the normal adult rat CNS: evidence for anterograde axonal transport. *J. Neurosci.* 17: 2295-2313.

Conti L, Cattaneo E. (2010) Neural stem cell system: physiological players or in vitro entities? *Nat. Rev. Neurosci.* 11: 176–187.

Curtis R, Adryan KM, Stark JL, Park JS, Compton DL, Weskamp G, Huber LJ, Chao MV, Jaenisch R, Lee KF, Lindsay RM, DiStefano PS. (1995) Differential role of the low affinity neurotrophin receptor (p75) in retrograde axonal transport of the neurotrophins. *Neuron* 14: 1201-1211.

Davies AM, Horton A, Burton LE, Schmelzer C, Vandlen R, Rosenthal A. (1993) Neurotrophin-4/5 is a mammalian-specific survival factor for distinct populations of sensory neurons. *J. Neurosci.* 13: 4961-4967.

Dechant G, Barde YA (2002) The neurotrophin receptor p75(NTR): novel functions and implications for diseases of the nervous system. *Nat. Neurosci.* 5: 1131-1136.

Delmaire C, Dumas EM, Sharman MA, van den Bogaard SJ, Valabregue R, Jauffret C, Justo D, Reilmann R, Stout JC, Craufurd D, Tabrizi SJ, Roos RA, Durr A, Lehéricy S. (2012) The structural correlates of functional deficits in early huntington's disease. *Hum. Brain Mapp.* [Electronic publication ahead of print].

del Toro D, Canals JM, Gines S, Kojima M, Egea G, Alberch J. (2006) Mutant huntingtin impairs the post-Golgi trafficking of brain-derived neurotrophic factor but not its Val66Met polymorphism. *J. Neurosci.* 26: 12748-12757.

DiFiglia M, Sapp E, Chase KO, Davies SW, Bates GP, Vonsattel JP, Aronin N. (1997) Aggregation of huntingtin in neuronal intranuclear inclusions and dystrophic neurites in brain. *Science* 277: 1990-1993.

DiFiglia M, Sapp E, Chase K, Schwarz C, Meloni A, Young C, Martin E, Vonsattel JP, Carraway R, Reeves SA, Boyce FM, Aronin N. (1995) Huntingtin is a cytoplasmic protein associated with vesicles in human and rat brain neurons. *Neuron* 14: 1075-1081.

Diniz BS, Teixeira AL (2011) Brain-derived neurotrophic factor and Alzheimer's disease: physiopathology and beyond. *Neuromolecular. Med.* 13: 217-222.

Djoussé L, Knowlton B, Cupples LA, Marder K, Shoulson I, Myers RH. (2002) Weight loss in early stage of Huntington's disease. *Neurology* 59: 1325-1330.

Dobrowsky RT, Carter BD (2000) p75 neurotrophin receptor signaling: mechanisms for neurotrophic modulation of cell stress? *J. Neurosci. Res.* 61: 237-243.

Duan W, Guo Z, Mattson MP. (2001a) Brain-derived neurotrophic factor mediates an excitoprotective effect of dietary restriction in mice *J. Neurochem.* 76: 619-626.

Duan W, Guo Z, Jiang H, Ladenheim B, Xu X, Cadet JL, Mattson MP. (2004) Paroxetine retards disease onset and progression in Huntingtin mutant mice. *Ann. Neurol.* 55: 590–594.

Duan W, Guo Z, Jiang H, Ware M, Li XJ, Mattson MP. (2003) Dietary restriction normalizes glucose metabolism and BDNF levels, slows disease progression, increases survival in huntingtin mutant mice. *Proc. Natl. Acad. Sci. USA* 100: 2911–2916.

Duan W, Lee J, Guo Z, Mattson MP. (2001b) Dietary restriction stimulates BDNF production in the brain *J. Mol. Neurosci.* 16: 1-12.

Duan W, Peng Q, Masuda N, Ford E, Tryggestad E, Ladenheim B, Zhao M, Cadet JL, Wong J, Ross CA. (2008) Sertraline slows disease progression and increases neurogenesis in N171-82Q mouse model of Huntington's disease. *Neurobiol. Dis.* 30: 312–322.

Duman RS. (1998) Novel therapeutic approaches beyond the serotonin receptor. *Biol. Psychiatry* 44: 324–335.

Dumas EM, van den Bogaard SJ, Ruber ME, Reilman RR, Stout JC, Craufurd D, Hicks SL, Kennard C, Tabrizi SJ, van Buchem MA, van der Grond J, Roos RA. (2012) Early changes in white matter *Hum. Brain Mapp.* 33: 203-212.

Encinas M, Iglesias M, Llecha N, Comella JX (1999) Extracellular-regulated kinases and phosphatidylinositol 3-kinase are involved in brain-derived neurotrophic factor-mediated survival and neuritogenesis of the neuroblastoma cell line SH-SY5Y. *J. Neurochem.* 73: 1409-1421.

Engelender S, Sharp AH, Colomer V, Tokito MK, Lanahan A, Worley P, Holzbaur EL, Ross CA. (1997) Huntingtin-associated protein 1 (HAP1) interacts with the p150Glued subunit of dynactin. *Hum. Mol. Genet.* 6: 2205-2212.

Farrer LA. (1985) Diabetes mellitus in Huntington disease. *Clin. Genet.* 27: 62-67.

Ferrer I, Goutan E, Marin C, Rey MJ, Ribalta T. (2000) Brain-derived neurotrophic factor in Huntington disease. *Brain Res.* 866: 257–261.

Frim DM, Uhler TA, Short MP, Ezzedine ZD, Klagsbrun M, Breakefield XO, Isacson O. (1993) Effects of biologically delivered NGF, BDNF and bFGF on striatal excitotoxic lesions. *Neuroreport* 4: 367–370.

Fox JH, Barber DS, Singh B, Zucker B, Swindell MK, Norflus F, Buzescu R, Chopra R, Ferrante RJ, Kazantsev A, Hersch SM. (2004) Cystamine increases L-cysteine levels in Huntington's disease transgenic mouse brain and in a PC12 model of polyglutamine aggregation. *J. Neurochem.* 91: 413–422.

Gauthier LR, Charrin BC, Borrell-Pages M, Dompierre JP, Rangone H, Cordelières FP, De Mey J, MacDonald ME, Lessmann V, Humbert S, Saudou F. (2004) Huntingtin controls neurotrophic support and survival of neurons by enhancing BDNF vesicular transport along microtubules. *Cell* 118: 127-138.

Gewirtz JC, Chen AC, Terwilliger R, Duman RC, Marek GJ. (2002) Modulation of DOI-induced increases in cortical BDNF expression by group II mGlu receptors. *Pharmacol. Biochem. Behav.* 73: 317–326.

Gharami K, Xie Y, An JJ, Tonegawa S, Xu B (2008) Brain-derived neurotrophic factor over-expression in the forebrain ameliorates Huntington's disease phenotypes in mice. *J. Neurochem.* 105: 369-379.

Gil JM, Leist M, Popovic N, Brundin P, Petersén A. (2004) Asialoerythropoietin is not effective in the R6/2 line of Huntington's disease mice. *BMC Neurosci.* 5: 17.

Gil JM, Mohapel P, Araújo IM, Popovic N, Li JY, Brundin P, Petersén A. (2005) Reduced hippocampal neurogenesis in R6/2 transgenic Huntington's disease mice. *Neurobiol. Dis.* 20: 744-751.

Gil JM, Rego AC. (2008) Mechanisms of neurodegeneration in Huntington's disease. *Eur. J. Neurosci.* 27: 2803-2820.

Gil JM, Rego AC. (2009) The R6 lines of transgenic mice: a model for screening new therapies for Huntington's disease. *Brain Res. Rev.* 59: 410-431.

Gill SS, Patel NK, Hotton GR, O'Sullivan K, McCarter R, Bunnage M, Brooks DJ, Svendsen CN, Heywood P. (2003) Direct brain infusion of glial cell line-derived neurotrophic factor in Parkinson disease. *Nat. Med.* 9: 589–595.

Gil-Mohapel JM. (2012) Screening of Therapeutic Strategies for Huntington's Disease in YAC128 Transgenic Mice. *CNS Neurosci. Ther.* 18: 77-86.

Gil-Mohapel J, Simpson JM, Christie BR. (2010) Modulation of adult neurogenesis by physical exercise and environmental enrichment: Insights for the treatment of neurological disorders. *Nervous System Diseases* Vol.1, Kunlin J (Eds). Transworld Research Network, Kerala, India, 125-150.

Gines S, Seong IS, Fossale E, Ivanova E, Trettel F, Gusella JF, Wheeler VC, Persichetti F, MacDonald ME. (2003) Specific progressive cAMP reduction implicates energy deficit in presymptomatic Huntington's disease knock-in mice. *Hum. Mol. Genet.* 12: 497–508.

Gray M, Shirasaki DI, Cepeda C, André VM, Wilburn B, Lu XH, Tao J, Yamazaki I, Li SH, Sun YE, Li XJ, Levine MS, Yang XW. (2008) Full-length human *J. Neurosci.* 28: 6182-6195.

Greenberg ME, Xu B, Lu B, Hempstead BL (2009) New insights in the biology of BDNF synthesis and release: implications in CNS function. *J. Neurosci.* 29: 12764-12767.

Grote HE, Bull ND, Howard ML, van Dellen A, Blakemore C, Bartlett PF, Hannan AJ. (2005) Cognitive disorders and neurogenesis deficits in Huntington's disease mice are rescued by fluoxetine. *Eur. J. Neurosci.* 22: 2081-2088.

Gunawardena S, Her LS, Brusch RG, Laymon RA, Niesman IR, Gordesky-Gold B, Sintasath L, Bonini NM, Goldstein LS. (2003) Disruption of axonal transport by loss of huntingtin or expression of pathogenic polyQ proteins in Drosophila. *Neuron* 40: 25-40.

Hacein-Bey-Abina S, Garrigue A, Wang GP, Soulier J, Lim A, Morillon E, Clappier E, Caccavelli L, Delabesse E, Beldjord K, Asnafi V, MacIntyre E, Dal Cortivo L, Radford I, Brousse N, Sigaux F, Moshous D, Hauer J, Borkhardt A, Belohradsky BH, Wintergerst U, Velez MC, Leiva L, Sorensen R, Wulffraat N, Blanche S, Bushman FD, Fischer A, Cavazzana-Calvo M. (2008) Insertional oncogenesis in 4 patients after retrovirus-mediated gene therapy of SCID-X1. *J. Clin. Invest.* 118: 3132–3142.

Hayden MR. (2000) Predictive testing for Huntington's disease: the calm after the storm. *Lancet.* 356: 1944-1945.

Hermel E, Gafni J, Propp SS, Leavitt BR, Wellington CL, Young JE, Hackam AS, Logvinova AV, Peel AL, Chen SF, Hook V, Singaraja R, Krajewski S, Goldsmith PC, Ellerby HM, Hayden MR, Bredesen DE, Ellerby LM. (2004) Specific caspase interactions and amplification are involved in selective neuronal vulnerability in Huntington's disease. *Cell Death Differ* 11: 424-438.

Heuser IJ, Chase TN, Mouradian MM. (1991) The limbic-hypothalamic-pituitary-adrenal axis in Huntington's disease. *Biol. Psychiatry* 30: 943-952.

Hobbs NZ, Pedrick AV, Say MJ, Frost C, Dar Santos R, Coleman A, Sturrock A, Craufurd D, Stout JC, Leavitt BR, Barnes J, Tabrizi SJ, Scahill RI. (2011) The structural involvement of the cingulate cortex *Mov. Disord.* 26: 1684-1690.

Hockly E, Cordery PM, Woodman B, Mahal A, van Dellen A, Blakemore C, Lewis CM, Hannan AJ, Bates GP. (2002) Environmental enrichment slows disease progression in R6/2 Huntington's disease mice. *Ann. Neurol.* 51: 235-242.

Hockly E, Tse J, Barker AL, Moolman DL, Beunard JL, Revington AP, Holt K, Sunshine S, Moffitt H, Sathasivam K, Woodman B, Wanker EE, Lowden PA, Bates GP. (2006) Evaluation of the benzothiazole aggregation inhibitors riluzole and PGL-135 as therapeutics for Huntington's disease. *Neurobiol. Dis.* 21: 228-236.

Hodgson JG, Agopyan N, Gutekunst CA, Leavitt BR, LePiane F, Singaraja R, Smith DJ, Bissada N, McCutcheon K, Nasir J, Jamot L, Li XJ, Stevens ME, Rosemond E, Roder JC, Phillips AG, Rubin EM, Hersch SM, Hayden MR. (1999) A YAC mouse model for Huntington's disease with full-length mutant huntingtin, cytoplasmic toxicity, and selective striatal neurodegeneration. *Neuron* 23: 181-192.

Hofer M, Pagliusi SR, Hohn A, Leibrock J, Barde YA (1990) Regional distribution of brain-derived neurotrophic factor mRNA in the adult mouse brain. *EMBO J.* 9: 2459-2464.

Huang EJ, Reichardt LF. (2001) Annu. Rev. Neurosci. 24, 677–736. 2. Woo N. H., Teng H. K., Siao C. J., Chiaruttini C., Pang P. T., Milner T. A., Hempstead B. L., Lu B. (2005) *Nat. Neurosci.* 8, 1069–1077.

Huber SJ, Paulson GW. (1987) Memory impairment associated with progression of Huntington's disease. *Cortex* 23: 275-283.

Ickes BR, Pham TM, Sanders LA, Albeck DS, Mohammed AH, Granholm AC. (2000) Long-term environmental enrichment leads to regional increases in neurotrophin levels in rat brain Exp Neurol 164: 45-52.

Kassubek J, Juengling FD, Kioschies T, Henkel K, Karitzky J, Kramer B, Ecker D, Andrich J, Saft C, Kraus P, Aschoff AJ, Ludolph AC, Landwehrmeyer GB. (2004) Topography of cerebral atrophy in early Huntington's disease: a voxel based morphometric MRI study. *J. Neurol. Neurosurg. Psychiatry* 75: 213-220.

Kells AP, Fong DM, Dragunow M, During MJ, Young D, Connor B. (2004) AAV-mediated gene delivery of BDNF or GDNF is neuroprotective in a model of Huntington disease. *Mol. Ther.* 9: 682–688.

Kempermann G, Kuhn HG, Gage FH. (1997) More hippocampal neurons in adult mice living in an enriched environment. Nature 386: 493-495.

Kernie SG, Liebl DJ, Parada LF (2000) BDNF regulates eating behavior and locomotor activity in mice. *EMBO J.* 19: 1290-1300.

Kirkwood SC, Su JL, Conneally P, Foroud T. (2001) Progression of symptoms in the early and middle stages of Huntington disease. *Arch Neurol.* 58: 273-278.

Kohl Z, Kandasamy M, Winner B, Aigner R, Gross C, Couillard-Despres S, Bogdahn U, Aigner L, Winkler J. (2007) Physical activity fails to rescue hippocampal neurogenesis deficits in the R6/2 mouse model of Huntington's disease. *Brain Res.* 1155: 24-33.

Kossel AH, Cambridge SB, Wagner U, Bonhoeffer T (2001) A caged Ab reveals an immediate/instructive effect of BDNF during hippocampal synaptic potentiation. *Proc. Natl. Acad. Sci. U S A* 98: 14702-14707.

Kremer HP, Roos RA, Dingjan GM, Bots GT, Bruyn GW, Hofman MA. (1991) The hypothalamic lateral tuberal nucleus *Neurosci Lett.* 132: 101-104.

Kremer HP, Roos RA, Dingjan G, Marani, Bots GT. (1990) Atrophy of the hypothalamic lateral tuberal nucleus in Huntington's disease. *J. Neuropathol. Exp. Neurol.* 49: 371-382.

Labuschagne I, Jones R, Callaghan J, Whitehead D, Dumas EM, Say MJ, Hart EP, Justo D, Coleman A, Dar Santos RC, Frost C, Craufurd D, Tabrizi SJ, Stout JC; TRACK-HD Investigators. (2012) Emotional face recognition *Psychiatry Re.* 207:118-126.

Langbehn DR, Hayden MR, Paulsen JS, PREDICT-HD Investigators of the Huntington Study Group. (2010) CAG-repeat length and the age *Am. J Med. Genet. B Neuropsychiatr. Genet.* 153B: 397-408.

Lazic SE, Grote H, Armstrong RJ, Blakemore C, Hannan AJ, van Dellen A, Barker RA. (2004) Decreased hippocampal cell proliferation in R6/1 Huntington's mice. *Neuroreport* 15: 811-813.

Lazic SE, Grote HE, Blakemore C, Hannan AJ, van Dellen A, Phillips W, Barker RA. (2006) Neurogenesis in the R6/1 transgenic mouse model of Huntington's disease: effects of environmental enrichment. *Eur. J. Neurosci.* 23: 1829-1838.

Leblhuber F, Peichl M, Neubauer C, Reisecker F, Steinparz FX, Windhager E, Maschek W. (1995) Serum dehydroepiandrosterone and cortisol measurements in Huntington's chorea. *J. Neurol. Sci.* 132: 76-79.

Lee FS, Kim AH, Khursigara G, Chao MV (2001) The uniqueness of being a neurotrophin receptor. *Curr. Opin. Neurobiol.* 11: 281-286.

Lee J, Duan W, Long JM, Ingram DK, Mattson MP. (2000) Dietary restriction increases the number of newly generated neural cells, and induces BDNF expression, in the dentate gyrus of rats. *J. Mol. Neurosci.* 15: 99-108.

Lee J, Seroogy KB, Mattson MP. (2002) Dietary restriction enhances neurotrophin expression and neurogenesis *J. Neurochem.* 80: 539-547.

Lesort M, Lee M, Tucholski J, Johnson GV. (2003) Cystamine inhibits caspase activity. Implications for the treatment of polyglutamine disorders. *J. Biol. Chem.* 278: 3825–3830.

Lessmann V, Gottmann K, Malcangio M (2003) Neurotrophin secretion: current facts and future prospects. *Prog. Neurobiol.* 69: 341-374.

Levine ES, Crozier RA, Black IB, Plummer MR (1998) Brain-derived neurotrophic factor modulates hippocampal synaptic transmission by increasing N-methyl-D-aspartic acid receptor activity. *Proc. Natl Acad. Sci. U S A* 95: 10235-10239.

Levine ES, Dreyfus CF, Black IB, Plummer MR (1995) Brain-derived neurotrophic factor rapidly enhances synaptic transmission in hippocampal neurons via postsynaptic tyrosine kinase receptors. *Proc. Natl. Acad. Sci. U S A* 92: 8074-8077.

Li JY, Popovic N, Brundin P. (2005) The use of the R6 transgenic mouse models of Huntington's disease in attempts to develop novel therapeutic strategies. *NeuroRx.* 2: 447-464.

Lohof AM, Ip NY, Poo MM (1993) Potentiation of developing neuromuscular synapses by the neurotrophins NT-3 and BDNF. Nature 363: 350-353.

Luthi-Carter R, Hanson SA, Strand AD, Bergstrom DA, Chun W, Peters NL, Woods AM, Chan EY, Kooperberg C, Krainc D, Young AB, Tapscott SJ, Olson JM. (2002) Dysregulation of gene expression in the R6/2 model of polyglutamine disease: parallel changes in muscle and brain. *Hum. Mol. Genet.* 11: 1911–1926.

Makkerh JP, Ceni C, Auld DS, Vaillancourt F, Dorval G, Barker PA. (2005) p75 neurotrophin receptor reduces ligand-induced Trk receptor ubiquitination and delays Trk receptor internalization and degradation. *EMBO Rep.* 6: 936-941.

Mangiarini L, Sathasivam K, Seller M, Cozens B, Harper A, Hetherington C, Lawton M, Trottier Y, Lehrach H, Davies SW, Bates GP. (1996) Exon 1 of the HD Gene with an Expanded CAG Repeat Is Sufficient to Cause a Progressive Neurological Phenotype in Transgenic Mice. *Cell* 87: 493-506.

Markianos M, Panas M, Kalfakis N, Vassilopoulos D. (2005) Plasma testosterone in male patients with Huntington's disease: relations to severity of illness and dementia. *Ann. Neurol.* 57: 520-525.

Martinez-Serrano A, Bjorklund A. (1996) Protection of the neostriatum against excitotoxic damage by neurotrophin-producing, genetically modified neural stem cells. *J. Neurosci.* 16: 4604–4616.

Masana Y, Wanaka A, Kato H, Asai T, Tohyama M (1993) Localization of trkB mRNA in postnatal brain development. *J. Neurosci. Res.* 35: 468-479.

Matsumoto T, Rauskolb S, Polack M, Klose J, Kolbeck R, Korte M, Barde YA. (2008) Biosynthesis and processing of endogenous BDNF: CNS neurons store and secrete BDNF, not pro-BDNF. *Nat. Neurosci.* 11: 131-133.

Mattson MP (2008) Glutamate and neurotrophic factors in neuronal plasticity and disease. *Ann. N Y Acad. Sci.* 1144: 97-112.

McAllister AK (1999) Subplate neurons: a missing link among neurotrophins, activity, and ocular dominance plasticity? *Proc. Natl. Acad. Sci. U S A* 96: 13600-13602.

McGuire JR, Rong J, Li SH, Li XJ (2006) Interaction of Huntingtin-associated protein-1 with kinesin light chain: implications in intracellular trafficking in neurons. *J. Biol. Chem.* 281: 3552-3559.

Murphy KP, Carter RJ, Lione LA, Mangiarini L, Mahal A, Bates GP, Dunnett SB, Morton AJ. (2000) Abnormal synaptic plasticity and impaired spatial cognition in mice transgenic for exon 1 of the human Huntington's disease mutation. *J. Neurosci.* 20: 5115-5123.

Neeper SA, Gómez-Pinilla F, Choi J, Cotman CW. (1996) Physical activity increases mRNA *Brain Res.* 726: 49-56.

Neeper SA, Gómez-Pinilla F, Choi J, Cotman C. (1995) Exercise and brain *Nature* 373: 109.

Nithianantharajah J, Barkus C, Vijiaratnam N, Clement O, Hannan AJ. (2009) Modeling brain reserve: experience-dependent neuronal plasticity in healthy and Huntington's disease transgenic mice. *Am. J. Geriatr. Psychiatry* 17: 196-209.

Oliff HS, Berchtold NC, Isackson P, Cotman CW. (1998) Exercise-induced regulation of brain *Brain Res. Mol. Brain Res.* 61(1-2):147-153.

Olson AK, Eadie BD, Ernst C, Christie BR. (2006) Environmental enrichment and voluntary exercise massively increase neurogenesis in the adult hippocampus via dissociable pathways. *Hippocampus* 16: 250-260.

Panegyres PK. (2004) The contribution of the study of neurodegenerative disorders *QJM*. 97: 555-567.

Pang TY, Hannan AJ. (2013) Enhancement of cognitive function *Neuropharmacology* 64: 515-528.

Pang TY, Stam NC, Nithianantharajah J, Howard ML, Hannan AJ. (2006) Differential effects of voluntary physical exercise on behavioral and brain-derived neurotrophic factor expression deficits in Huntington's disease transgenic mice. *Neuroscience* 141: 569-584.

Pencea V, Bingaman KD, Wiegand SJ, Luskin MB. (2001) Infusion of brain-derived neurotrophic factor into the lateral ventricle of the adult rat leads to new neurons in the parenchyma of the striatum, septum, thalamus, and hypothalamus. *J. Neurosci.* 21: 6706-6717.

Peng Q, Masuda N, Jiang M, Li Q, Zhao M, Ross CA, Duan W. (2008) The antidepressant sertraline improves the phenotype, promotes neurogenesis and increases BDNF levels in the R6/2 Huntington's disease mouse model. *Exp. Neurol.* 210: 154-163.

Perez-Navarro E, Alberch J, Neveu I, Arenas E. (1999) Brain-derived neurotrophic factor, neurotrophin-3 and neurotrophin-4/5 differentially regulate the phenotype and prevent degenerative changes in striatal projection neurons after excitotoxicity in vivo. *Neuroscience* 91: 1257–1264.

Perez-Navarro E, Canudas AM, Akerund P, Alberch J, Arenas E. (2000) Brain-derived neurotrophic factor, neurotrophin-3, and neurotrophin-4/5 prevent the death of striatal projection neurons in a rodent model of Huntington's disease. *J. Neurochem.* 75: 2190–2199.

Petersen A, Bjorkqvist M. (2006) Hypothalamic-endocrine aspects in Huntington's disease. *Eur. J. Neurosci.* 24: 961-967.

Petersen A, Gil J, Maat-Schieman ML, Bjorkqvist M, Tanila H, Araújo IM, Smith R, Popovic N, Wierup N, Norlén P, Li JY, Roos RA, Sundler F, Mulder H, Brundin P. (2005) Orexin loss in Huntington's disease. *Hum. Mol. Genet.* 14: 39-47.

Pineda JR, Pardo R, Zala D, Yu H, Humbert S, Saudou F. (2009) Genetic and pharmacological inhibition of calcineurin corrects the BDNF transport defect in Huntington's disease. *Mol. Brain.* 2: 33.

Podolsky S, Leopold NA, Sax DS. (1972) Increased frequency of diabetes mellitus in patients with Huntington's chorea. *Lancet* 1: 1356-1358.

Pouladi MA, Graham RK, Karasinska JM, Xie Y, Santos RD, Petersén A, Hayden MR. (2009) Prevention of depressive behaviour in the YAC128 mouse model of Huntington disease by mutation at residue 586 of huntingtin. *Brain* 132: 919-932.

Powrozek TA, Sari Y, Singh RP, Zhou FC. (2004) Neurotransmitters and substances of abuse: Effects on adult neurogenesis. *Curr. Neurovasc. Res.* 1: 251–260.

Reichardt LF (2006) Neurotrophin-regulated signalling pathways. *Philos. Trans. R. Soc. Lond. B Biol. Sci.* 361: 1545-1564.

Reiner A, Wang HB, Del Mar N, Sakata K, Yoo W, Deng YP. (2012) BDNF may play a differential role in the protective effect of the mGluR2/3 agonist *Brain Res.* 1473: 161-72.

Rigamonti D, Bolognini D, Mutti C, Zuccato C, Tartari M, Sola F, Valenza M, Kazantsev AG, Cattaneo E. (2007) Loss of huntingtin function complemented by small molecules acting as repressor element 1/neuron restrictive silencer element silencer modulators. *J. Biol. Chem.* 282: 24554–24562.

Rosas HD, Koroshetz WJ, Chen YI, Skeuse C, Vangel M, Cudkowicz ME, Caplan K, Marek K, Seidman LJ, Makris N, Jenkins BG, Goldstein JM. (2003) Evidence for more widespread cerebral pathology in early HD: an MRI-based morphometric analysis. *Neurology* 60: 1615-1620.

Rossi F, Cattaneo E. (2002) Opinion: neural stem cell therapy for neurological diseases: dreams and reality. *Nat. Rev. Neurosci.* 3: 401–409.

Roux PP, Barker PA (2002) Neurotrophin signaling through the p75 neurotrophin receptor. *Prog. Neurobiol.* 67: 203-233.

Ryu JK, Kim J, Cho SJ, Hatori K, Nagai A, Choi HB, Lee MC, McLarnon JG, Kim SU. (2004) Proactive transplantation of human neural stem cells prevents degeneration of striatal neurons in a rat model of Huntington disease. *Neurobiol. Dis.* 16: 68–77.

Sanberg PR, Fibiger HC, Mark RF. (1981) Body weight and dietary factors in Huntington's disease patients compared with matched controls. *Med. J. Aust.* 1: 407-409.

Sari Y. (2011) Potential Drugs and Methods for Preventing or Delaying the Progression of Huntington's Disease. *Recent Pat. CNS Drug Discov.* 6(2):80-90.

Satomura E, Baba H, Nakano Y, Maeshima H, Suzuki T, Arai H. (2011) Correlations between brain-derived neurotrophic factor and clinical symptoms in medicated patients with major depression. *J. Affect. Disord.* 135: 332-335.

Say MJ, Jones R, Scahill RI, Dumas EM, Coleman A, Santos RC, Justo D, Campbell JC, Queller S, Shores EA, Tabrizi SJ, Stout JC; TRACK-HD Investigators. (2011) Visuomotor integration *Neuropsychologia* 49: 264-270.

Schiefer J, Landwehrmeyer GB, Luesse HG, Sprünken A, Puls C, Milkereit A, Milkereit E, Kosinski CM. (2002) Riluzole prolongs survival time and alters nuclear inclusion formation in a transgenic mouse model of Huntington's disease. *Mov. Disord.* 17: 748-757.

Schilling G, Becher MW, Sharp AH, Jinnah HA, Duan K, Kotzuk JA, Slunt HH, Ratovitski T, Cooper JK, Jenkins NA, Copeland NG, Price DL, Ross CA, Borchelt DR. (1999) Intranuclear inclusions and neuritic aggregates in transgenic mice expressing a mutant NH_2-terminal fragment of huntingtin. *Hum. Mol. Genet.* 8: 397–407.

Schilling G, Savonenko AV, Coonfield ML, Morton JL, Vorovich E, Gale A, Neslon C, Chan N, Eaton M, Fromholt D, Ross CA, Borchelt DR. (2004) Environmental, pharmacological, and genetic modulation of the HD phenotype in transgenic mice. *Exp. Neurol.* 187: 137-149.

Schmidtke K, Manner H, Kaufmann R, Schmolck H. (2002) Cognitive procedural learning in patients with fronto-striatal lesions. *Learn Mem.* 9: 419–429.

Simmons DA, Rex CS, Palmer L, Pandyarajan V, Fedulov V, Gall CM, Lynch G. (2009) Up-regulating BDNF with an ampakine rescues synaptic plasticity and memory in Huntington's disease knockin mice. *Proc. Natl. Acad. Sci. USA* 106: 4906–4911.

Simpson JM, Gil-Mohapel J, Pouladi MA, Ghilan M, Xie Y, Hayden MR, Christie BR. (2011) Altered adult hippocampal neurogenesis in the YAC128 transgenic mouse model of Huntington disease. *Neurobiol. Dis.* 41: 249-260.

Slaughter JR, Martens MP, Slaughter KA. (2001) Depression and Huntington's disease: prevalence, clinical manifestations, etiology, and treatment. *CNS Spectr.* 6: 306-326.

Slow EJ, van Raamsdonk J, Rogers D, Coleman SH, Graham RK, Deng Y, Oh R, Bissada N, Hossain SM, Yang YZ, Li XJ, Simpson EM, Gutekunst CA, Leavitt BR, Hayden MR. (2003) Selective striatal neuronal loss in a YAC128 mouse model of Huntington disease. *Hum. Mol. Genet.* 12: 1555-1567.

Soneson C, Fontes M, Zhou Y, Denisov V, Paulsen JS, Kirik D, Petersén A; Huntington Study Group PREDICT-HD investigators. (2010) Early changes in the hypothalamic region in prodromal Huntington disease revealed by MRI *Neurobiol. Dis.* 40: 531-543.

Spargo E, Everall IP, Lantos PL. (1993) Neuronal loss in the hippocampus in Huntington's disease: a comparison with HIV infection. *J. Neurol.Neurosurg. Psychiatry 56*: 487-491.

Spires TL, Grote HE, Garry S, Cordery PM, Van Dellen A, Blakemore C, Hannan AJ. (2004) Dendritic spine pathology and deficits in experience-dependent dendritic plasticity in R6/1 Huntington's disease transgenic mice. *Eur. J. Neurosci.* 19: 2799-2807.

Squitieri F, Orobello S, Cannella M, Martino T, Romanelli P, Giovacchini G, Frati L, Mansi L, Ciarmiello A. (2009) Riluzole protects Huntington disease patients from brain glucose hypometabolism and grey matter volume loss and increases production of neurotrophins. *Eur. J. Nucl. Med. Mol. Imaging* 36: 1113–1120.

Stout JC, Jones R, Labuschagne I, O'Regan AM, Say MJ, Dumas EM, Queller S, Justo D, Santos RD, Coleman A, Hart EP, Dürr A, Leavitt BR, Roos RA, Langbehn DR, Tabrizi SJ, Frost C. (2012) Evaluation *J. Neurol. Neurosurg. Psychiatry* 83: 687-694.

Strand AD, Baquet ZC, Aragaki AK, Holmans P, Yang L, Cleren C, Beal MF, Jones L, Kooperberg C, Olson JM, Jones KR. (2007) Expression profiling of Huntington's disease model *J. Neurosci.* 27: 11758-11768.

Sullivan FR, Bird ED, Alpay M, Cha JH. (2001) Remotivation therapy and Huntington's disease. *J. Neurosci. Nurs*. 33: 136–142.

Tabrizi SJ, Scahill RI, Durr A, Roos RA, Leavitt BR, Jones R, Landwehrmeyer GB, Fox, Johnson H, Hicks SL, Kennard C, Craufurd D, Frost C, Langbehn DR, Reilmann R, Stout JC; TRACK-HD Investigators. (2011) Biological and clinical changes in premanifest and early stage Huntington's disease in the TRACK-HD study: the 12-month longitudinal analysis. *Lancet Neurol*. 10: 31-42.

Teixeira AL, Barbosa IG, Diniz BS, Kummer A (2010) Circulating levels of brain-derived neurotrophic factor: correlation with mood, cognition and motor function. *Biomark Med*. 4: 871-887.

Teng HK, Teng KK, Lee R, Wright S, Tevar S, Almeida RD, Kermani P, Torkin R, Chen ZY, Lee FS, Kraemer RT, Nykjaer A, Hempstead BL. (2005) ProBDNF induces neuronal apoptosis via activation of a receptor complex of p75NTR and sortilin. *J. Neurosci.* 25: 5455-5463.

The Huntington's Disease Collaborative Research Group. (1993) A novel gene containing a trinucleotide repeat that is expanded and unstable on Huntington's disease chromosomes. *Cell* 72: 971-983.

Thomas K, Davies A (2005) Neurotrophins: a ticket to ride for BDNF. *Curr. Biol.* 15: R262-264.

Vaidya VA, Marek GJ, Aghajanian GK, Duman RS. (1997) 5-HT2A receptor-mediated regulation of brain-derived neurotrophic factor mRNA in the hippocampus and the neocortex. *J. Neurosci.* 17: 2785–2795.

Vaidya VA, Terwilliger RM, Duman RS. (1999) Role of 5-HT2A receptors in the stress-induced down-regulation of brain-derived neurotrophic factor expression in rat hippocampus. *Neurosci. Lett.* 262:1–4.

van Dellen A, Blakemore C, Deacon R, York D, Hannan AJ. (2000) Delaying the onset of Huntington's in mice. *Nature* 404: 721-722.

van Dellen A, Cordery PM, Spires TL, Blakemore C, Hannan AJ. (2008) Wheel running from a juvenile age delays onset of specific motor deficits but does not alter protein aggregate density in a mouse model of Huntington's disease. *BMC Neurosci.* 9: 34.

Van Praag H, Christie BR, Sejnowski TJ, Gage FH. (1999a) Running enhances neurogenesis, learning, and long-term potentiation in mice. *Proc. Natl. Acad. Sci. USA* 96: 13427-13431.

Van Praag H, Kempermann G, Gage FH. (1999b) Running increases cell proliferation and neurogenesis in the adult mouse dentate gyrus. *Nat. Neurosci.* 2: 266-270.

Van Raamsdonk JM, Pearson J, Slow EJ, Hossain SM, Leavitt BR, Hayden MR. (2005) Cognitive dysfunction precedes neuropathology and motor abnormalities in the YAC128 mouse model of Huntington's disease. *J. Neurosci.* 25: 4169-4180.

Vonsattel JP, DiFiglia M. (1998) Huntington disease. *J. Neuropathol. Exp. Neurol.* 57: 369-384.

Waterhouse EG, Xu B (2009) New insights into the role of brain-derived neurotrophic factor in synaptic plasticity. *Mol. Cell Neurosci.* 42: 81-89.

Webb M, Trzepacz PT. (1987) Huntington's disease: correlations of mental status with chorea. *Biol. Psychiatry* 22: 751-761.

Wolf RC, Grön G, Sambataro F, Vasic N, Wolf ND, Thomann PA, Saft C, Landwehrmeyer GB, Orth M. (2011) Magnetic resonance perfusion *J. Cereb. Blood Flow Metab.* 31: 1908-1918.

Woo NH, Teng HK, Siao CJ, Chiaruttini C, Pang PT, Milner TA, Hempstead BL, Lu B. (2005) Activation of p75NTR by proBDNF facilitates hippocampal long-term depression. *Nat. Neurosci.* 8: 1069-1077.

Xu H, Steven Richardson J, Li XM (2003) Dose-related effects of chronic antidepressants on neuroprotective proteins BDNF, Bcl-2 and Cu/Zn-SOD in rat hippocampus. *Neuropsychopharmacology* 28: 53-62.

Yan Q, Rosenfeld RD, Matheson CR, Hawkins N, Lopez OT, Bennett L, Welcher AA. (1997) Expression of brain-derived neurotrophic factor protein in the adult rat central nervous system. *Neuroscience* 78: 431-448.

Yanez-Munoz RJ, Balaggan KS, MacNeil A, Howe SJ, Schmidt M, Smith AJ, Buch P, MacLaren RE, Anderson PN, Barker SE, Duran Y, Bartholomae C, von Kalle C, Heckenlively JR, Kinnon C, Ali RR, Thrasher AJ. (2006) Effective gene therapy with nonintegrating lentiviral vectors. *Nat. Med.* 12: 348–353.

Yoshii A, Constantine-Paton M (2010) Postsynaptic BDNF-TrkB signaling in synapse maturation, plasticity, and disease. Dev Neurobiol 70: 304-322.

Young D, Lawlor PA, Leone P, Dragunow M, During MJ. (1999) Environmental enrichment inhibits spontaneous apoptosis *Nat. Med.* 5: 448-453.

Zajac MS, Pang TY, Wong N, Weinrich B, Leang LS, Craig JM, Saffery R, Hannan AJ. (2010) Wheel running and environmental enrichment differentially modify exon-specific BDNF expression in the hippocampus of wild-type and pre-motor symptomatic male and female Huntington's disease mice. *Hippocampus* 20: 621-636.

Zhang Y, Li M, Drozda M, Chen M, Ren S, Mejia Sanchez RO, Leavitt BR, Cattaneo E, Ferrante RJ, Hayden MR, Friedlander RM. (2003) Depletion of wild-type huntingtin in mouse models of neurologic diseases. *J. Neurochem.* 87: 101–106.

Zigova T, Pencea V, Wiegand SJ, Luskin MB. (1998) Intraventricular administration of BDNF increases the number of newly generated neurons in the adult olfactory bulb. *Mol. Cell Neurosci.* 11: 234-245.

Zuccato C, Cattaneo E (2007) Role of brain-derived neurotrophic factor in Huntington's disease. *Prog. Neurobiol.* 81: 294-330.

Zuccato C, Ciammola A, Rigamonti D, Leavitt BR, Goffredo D, Conti L, MacDonald ME, Friedlander RM, Silani V, Hayden MR, Timmusk T,

Sipione S, Cattaneo E. (2001) Loss of huntingtin-mediated BDNF gene transcription in Huntington's disease. *Science* 293: 493-498.

Zuccato C, Liber D, Ramos C, Tarditi A, Rigamonti D, Tartari M, Valenza M, Cattaneo E. (2005) Progressive loss of BDNF in a mouse model of Huntington's disease and rescue by BDNF delivery. *Pharmacol. Res.* 52: 133–139.

Zuccato C, Marullo M, Vitali B, Tarditi A, Mariotti C, Valenza M, Lahiri N, Wild EJ, Sassone J, Ciammola A, Bachoud-Lèvi AC, Tabrizi SJ, Di Donato S, Cattaneo E. (2011) Brain-derived neurotrophic factor in patients with Huntington's disease. *PLoS One*. 2011;6(8):e22966.

Zuccato C, Tartari M, Crotti A, Goffredo D, Valenza M, Conti L, Cataudella T, Leavitt BR, Hayden MR, Timmusk T, Rigamonti D, Cattaneo E. (2003) Huntingtin interacts with RES *Nat. Genet.* 35: 76-83.

Zuccato C, Valenza M, Cattaneo E. (2010) Molecular mechanisms and potential therapeutical targets in Huntington's disease. *Physiol. Rev.* 90: 905-981.

In: Huntington's Disease
Editors: K. Guillory, A. M. Carrasco
ISBN: 978-1-62808-316-3

Chapter III

The Legal Ramifications of Huntington's Disease

Ian Freckelton
Barrister, Crockett Chambers, Melbourne, Australia; Professorial Fellow, Melbourne Law School and Department of Psychiatry, Faculty of Medicine, Dentistry and Health Sciences, University of Melbourne, Australia

Author's Note

The author acknowledges the helpful suggestions of Dr Patricia Molloy. The chapter draws upon and updates material in I Freckelton, "Huntington's Disease and the Law" (2010) 18 *Journal of Law and Medicine* 7-18 and was written while the author was staying in Langford Budville in Somerset. It is written in memory of the late Captain John Lloyd.

Abstract

Huntington's disease (HD) has serious and disabling mental as well as physical effects, in particular symptoms of depression, impulsivity and paranoia. Such symptoms impact upon those who have HD, those with the potential to inherit it, and those who care for and are close to persons with HD. The symptoms can have many legal ramifications, including in relation to evolving impairments of capacity which can have an outcome in terms of involuntary status as mental health patients, testamentary capacity and the need for guardianship and administration orders. The evolving disease can have effects upon fitness for parenting, obligations to pay spousal and child maintenance, and the quantum of compensation from a tortious incident to which a person is entitled. It can have repercussions for criminal liability and culpability. This chapter reviews case law from a number of countries in relation to such matters, noting the broader radiation to relatives and carers of the effects of HD, and reflecting on the need for legal and medical professionals to be aware of the legal consequences of HD so that they can discharge their responsibilities holistically, sensitively and informedly.

Introduction

Aside from its physical symptomatology which, amongst other things, is characterised by distinctive choreic (writhing) movements [1], adversely affected gait and a reduced capacity to swallow, Huntington's Disease ("HD") produces impaired executive functioning and a host of affective symptoms which can mimic psychotic and dementing conditions. A consequence is that HD has the potential for multiple legal ramifications for those diagnosed with the disease or at risk of contracting it.

HD was identified as a focus of United States eugenics research and debate in the 1920s and 1930s [2] and then singled out legislatively for eugenic extermination by the Nazis along with other inherited and congenital conditions that were seen to weaken the gene pool [3]. Article I of the *Law for the Prevention of Genetically Diseased Offspring 1933* (Ger) defined who was to be examined and then sterilized by order of courts constituted for making such decisions:

1) Anyone who suffers from an inheritable disease may be surgically sterilized if, in the judgement of medical science, it could be expected that his descendants will suffer from serious inherited mental or physical defects.
2) Anyone who suffers from one of the following is to be regarded as inheritably diseased within the meaning of this law:
    a) congenital feeble-mindedness
    b) schizophrenia
    c) manic-depression

d) congenital epilepsy
e) inheritable St Vitus' dance (Huntington's Chorea)
f) hereditary blindness
g) hereditary deafness
h) serious inheritable malformations [4].

Commencing during this period, but persisting to this day, a major issue in relation to HD is discrimination and genetic stigmatization, including in employment, access to insurance for those with HD, entitlement to social security [5], within social relationships and during a range of ordinary encounters [6].

This chapter explores a range of areas that legal decision-making in a number of countries has identified as having a relevance for HD in terms of administrative, discrimination, criminal, civil and family law litigation. It selects cases to illustrate a cross-section of relevant legal issues for persons with HD or at risk of developing it. It argues that HD constitutes one of a number of areas of pathology about which greater awareness is needed within the legal system so as more informedly to inform court and tribunal processes. This is also necessary so that protections are effectively accorded to those with HD, those at risk of becoming symptomatic with it and those who live and care for persons with HD.

Clinical Issues Relevant to the Law

There is much that remains to be learned about the pathology and genetics of HD in spite of important strides in our knowledge during the latter part of the twentieth century and early in the twenty first. Although HD is known to be caused by a CAG (cytosine, adenine, guanine) trinucleotide expansion in the first exon of the HD gene [7] and although the HD gene was mapped to chromosome 4 in 1983 and cloned in 1993, as yet this has provided little practical assistance for persons diagnosed as being at risk of becoming symptomatic with it.

The HD codes for production of a protein called "huntingtin," but the protein's function is still unknown. The altered huntingtin protein contains many more molecules of the amino than regular huntingtin because of repetitive copies of the CAG codon in the Huntington gene [8]. However, it remains to be determined whether NIs are a cause a result of HD or a defence mechanism against it [9].

The structure of the CAG repeat is important for prediction of those who will ultimately contract the disease. It is highly polymorphic and varies from 6 to 37 repeats on chromosomes of unaffected individuals and from more than 30 to 180 repeats on chromosomes of those with HD [10]. Persons with 28 or fewer repeats will not develop HD; nor will their children. Those with more than 40 generally will develop HD and their children have a 50% chance of doing so. However, there is an area of uncertainty: "It appears that people who have 29–35 repeats will not develop HD themselves, but a small percentage of their children may. People with repeats in the range of 36 to 39 are considered to be in a 'grey zone'; they may or may not develop HD and, likewise, their children may or may not be affected by the mutant gene [11]." This frequently engenders particular distress, anxiety and depression and in itself has been criminogenic in terms of behaviours arising from the stress of uncertainty.

Characteristic neuropathology in HD occurs within the neostriatum or striate nucleus (a subcortical part of the forebrain), in which gross atrophy of the caudate nucleus and putamen [12] is accompanied by selective neuronal loss and astrogliosis, an abnormal increase in the number of astrocytes due to the destruction of nearby neurons. Marked neuronal loss is also identifiable in deep layers of the cerebral cortex. Other regions, including the globus pallidus, thalamus, subthalamic nucleus, substantia nigra, and cerebellum, show varying degrees of atrophy depending on the stage of a patient's development of HD [13].

The result is that HD has many health and therefore legal consequences. Amongst other things, it causes uncontrolled movements, deterioration of cognitive function, and emotional disturbance. It can affect co-ordination, thought, perception, and memory. It is well known that many with HD experience involuntary movements of the arms, legs, body, and face (chorea). However, less recognized is that often these symptoms are often accompanied by affective lability, depression, impulsivity, irritability, slurred speech, and clumsiness [14]. There are new indications that the depression suffered by many with HD may be glutamate-based [15].

HD manifests in its early phase in erratic mood, depression, irritability, and difficulties in learning new information, remembering a fact, or making a decision. Quarrell [16] stresses this aspect of the disease, observing that "many families find it more difficult to cope with the wide range of behavioural and emotional problems than with the physical aspects of the condition". As the disease progresses, concentration on intellectual tasks becomes increasingly difficult and the patient may have difficulty feeding himself or herself and in swallowing. Many display considerable apathy, partly arising from depression.

There is a high incidence of suicide amongst those with HD [17], including those who are prodromal [18]; in a 2011 study [19] of 1941 HD patients, 19% (n=369) endorsed suicidal ideation, leading the authors to recommend routine suicidality assessment for those diagnosed with HD.

The rate of disease progression and the age of onset vary from person to person. When the disease progresses, a variety of symptoms emerge, including increasing problems in swallowing, loss of balance (ataxia), impaired reasoning, and memory problems. It is important to observe that HD is a progressive condition that affects people differently, often quite slowly, leading to a significant incidence of misdiagnosis in its early phases. A person with HD may live for 15 to 25 years after developing the first symptoms [20]. Death is commonly caused by a complication of the disease such as choking, or an injury related to a fall. In the period leading toward death, HD may impact upon whether a person is able to take the physical steps necessary to terminate their own life [21]. Fear of cognitive decline, of total dependency, and being unable to find meaning in life, have been found to be important issues for HD patients in a study in the Netherlands related to euthanasia sought by those with HD [22].

Each child of an HD parent has a 50-50 chance of inheriting the HD gene [23]. When a child does not inherit the HD gene, he or she will not develop the disease and cannot pass it to subsequent generations but for those who inherit the HD gene it is a matter of time until they develop the disease. Whether one child within a family inherits the gene has no bearing on whether others will or will not inherit it. In between 1 and 3 percent of those ultimately diagnosed with HD, no family history of HD is found.

Generally, though, HD has an adult onset with its mean age of commencement of symptoms being 40 years but in 5 to 10% of cases its symptoms commence in persons under 20 years of age [24]. The symptoms of the juvenile form of HD, or "Westphal variant", are somewhat different from adult-onset HD: "Initial symptoms usually involve slow, stiff and awkward walking and talking, choking, clumsiness and falling. Later, the child may become slow to respond and performance at school may become erratic. The course of the juvenile form is generally more rapid than the adult-onset HD [25]."

In the United States about 30,000 people have HD, while some 200,000 are at risk of contracting it [26]. In addition, 35,000 people exhibit some symptoms and 75,000 people carry the abnormal gene that will cause them to develop the disease [27]. In the United Kingdom there are between 4,200 and 6,000 patients with HD at any time [28]. The incidence of HD is somewhat variable across different populations with the Lake Maracaibo region in Venezuela being 700 per 100,000 people, the island of Mauritius 46 per 100,000 people, and Tasmania in Australia 17.4 per 100,000 people [29]. The prevalence in most European countries ranges from 1.63-9.95 per 100,000 people but the prevalence of HD in Finland and Japan is less than 1 per 100,000 people [30].

Treatment of HD (there being no cure as yet) targets different aspects of its symptomatology, including involuntary movements, psychosis, depression, anxiety and swallowing difficulties. A number of drugs are also prescribed to address emotional and movement problems associated with HD. In August 2008 the United States Food and Drug Administration approved tetrabenazine to treat Huntington's chorea (the involuntary writhing movements), making it the first drug approved for use in the United States specifically to treat the disease. Most drugs used to treat the symptoms of HD have side-effects such as fatigue, restlessness, or hyperexcitability. However, for the present it is only symptoms that are treated.

A number of such treatable symptoms are psychiatric with depression and anxiety being common, as well as (less often) irritability and aggression [31]. Treatments for HD without any evidence base have been promoted by the unscrupulous, resulting, for instance, in *Commissioner for Fair Trading, Department of Commerce v Perrett* [2007] NSWSC 1130 in determinations that spurious representations about substances distributed to address the symptoms of HD were misleading and deceptive and thus unlawful.

There are three forms of testing for HD [32]: presymptomatic for those at risk but not showing symptoms; confirmatory for those exhibiting possible symptoms; and prenatal testing to determine whether a foetus is at risk for HD. The testing has a very high right of accuracy. The existence of such testing options raises a range of ethical legal and insurance issues.

In particular, the psychiatric symptomatology that often accompanies the degenerative phases of HD has relevance in law [33] and ethics [34] for insurance purposes [35], testamentary capacity (and the making of wills while there is such capacity) [36], involuntary status under mental health legislation, guardianship and administration orders, family law responsibilities and even entitlement for compensation if a personal intervenes.

HD and Insurance

The potential for discrimination against persons with HD is particularly high in the insurance context. Fear of health insurance discrimination has been identified to be a strong motive in refraining from obtaining genetic testing [37]. In the United States a number of steps have been taken to reduce this risk. They are of particular application to persons with HD.

In May 2008, the updated *Genetic Information Nondiscrimination Act* (US) (GINA) was signed into federal law with many of its provisions coming into effect by May 2010. It prohibits health insurers and employers from discriminating against a person based on genetic information, a term which is broadly defined. An aim of the legislation is to provide that no one can be denied insurance or charged a higher premium based on genetic information, and that health insurance companies cannot request genetic information from any person or their family members. In addition, it precludes employers making decisions about hiring, firing, or promotion based on genetic information. However, importantly, GINA does not apply to life insurance, disability insurance, long-term care insurance, and employers with fewer than 15 employees.

Under the *Affordable Care Act 2010* (US), adults with existing disabilities and mental or physical illnesses cannot be denied health insurance coverage as of 1 January 2014.

Imposition of Involuntary Status

HD is not itself a mental illness but, as noted above, it gives rise first to impaired executive functions and then quite regularly to paranoid ideation and to dementia-like symptoms which can constitute significant disturbances to thought, capacity for rational thought or thought form, stream of thought, and memory, often resulting in limited capacity on the part of the person to consent to needed psychical and psychiatric treatment, and thus a risk to the health and safety of the person and, sometimes, to others. This means that in some jurisdictions the criteria for involuntary status, either as a mandated inpatient or outpatient in the community may be satisfied. In all countries the key questions in this regard are the extent to which the symptoms require treatment and the risk being posed to the person or others by the symptoms that are being experienced by reason of the HD. Inevitably the person's insight into their degenerative conditions and its consequences for them impact upon both the likelihood of their complying with needed treatment and their ability to consent to it.

For clinicians and mental healthcare and capacity tribunals determining whether a person should be made involuntary HD gives rise to a number of challenges. These range from clear identification of the disorder to overlaps in its symptomatology with other conditions with which it may be confused.

In *Re CS* 2011 CanLII 34999 (ON CCB), for instance, the patient, CS, was a woman of above average intelligence in her 40s. She had HD. She had been showing increasing signs of dementia and frontal lobe dysfunction, which in turn had resulted in her neglecting her personal care and failing to eat adequately. While in hospital, she regained some weight and attended more consistently to her personal hygiene. However, not long after being discharged into the community, in spite of intensive follow-up by a treatment team and a community psychiatrist, CS lost approximately sixteen pounds in six weeks and was found by once again to be living in dangerously unsanitary conditions. Her attending physician sought to place her on anti-psychotic medications but she refused. At this point, her physician found CS incapable of consenting to treatment with anti-psychotics and made her an involuntary patient. CS applied to the Ontario Consent and Capacity Board for a review of the finding of her incapacity to consent to treatment and her involuntary detention.

The Board accepted the physician's assertion that CS lacked insight into the nature of her illness, the manifestations of her dementia and the likely consequences of failing to care for herself by eating adequately. It found that because she did not appreciate that she had a mental disorder, CS was not able to see the risks and benefits of taking medication aimed to ameliorate the effects of the disorder. Nor was she able to appreciate the risks and benefits of a decision not to take medication that could ameliorate her mental disorder. It confirmed the finding of incapacity with respect to the proposed treatment on the basis that CS was unable by reason of HD to appreciate the reasonably foreseeable consequences of a decision or lack of decision about the treatment in question, anti-psychotic medications.

The needs of a person in advanced HD were highlighted in *Re DM*, 2011 CanLII 70531 (ON CCB) where the patient, DM, was 55 years of age with dementia due to advanced Huntington's Disease. DM had been a palliative care patient at the Hospital since 2009. He had minimal motor coordination and could not walk or communicate. It was not disputed that DM did not "belong" in a psychiatric hospital, and would be better suited for care in an appropriate long-term care facility; however, practically speaking, there was nowhere else for DM to go. Very few healthcare facilities were willing or able to provide the level of care required for a person with advanced HD. DM required physical restraints and continuous care but no long-term care facility was willing or able to take him.

The Board accepted that without being able to restrain DM physically, staff could not prevent DM from sustaining serious injury from falling or striking out at an object or staff person due to chorea. Without continuous nursing care available at the hospital, DM would not be able to feed himself, go to the toilet, brush his teeth, or even sit up. Nursing care was needed to help him get in and out of bed, in and out of his chair, and to walk without injury. Without nursing care, DM would be not be able to survive, and would suffer both substantial physical deterioration and grave physical impairment.

The Board found that DM was incapable of consenting to treatment, that he could not be treated as a voluntary patient and that it was likely he would suffer serious physical impairment/ substantial physical deterioration if not treated, and if he was not required to remain at the hospital. It concluded that if DM were to leave the hospital, it would be unlikely that he would be able to survive, as the level of care required was not available: he needed a variety of treatments, including pharmacotherapy, which he could not take on his own, as well as the care prescribed by the nursing staff for therapeutic, preventative and palliative purposes. Thus, it confirmed the involuntary order in relation to him.

The situation with patients with HD is not static and can yield quite different outcomes at different junctures in the progression of the disease. In *Re B*, 2009 Can LII 47221 (ON CCB), a hearing took place in relation to a patient, B, who was a 52 year old woman who had appeared before the Ontario Consent and Capacity Board on six occasions since 2008. Her HD was "declining" and she had lost her capacity to care for herself and been found incapable to consent to long term care. A neurologist stated in a report that "Disturbances of cognition are characterized by memory loss, anosognosia (lack of self-awareness), loss of cognitive speed and poor judgment. Difficulties are apparent in the person's ability to plan, organize, prioritize and initiate. Because these executive functions are no longer intact, the person with HD loses the ability to problem-solve and to judge situations appropriately. Normal day-to-day activity also becomes difficult because, quite quickly after the onset of symptoms, the ability to think sequentially becomes impaired." However, the Board found there to be "no objective or even substantive evidence of cognitive decline, or in fact mental disorder". As the onus was not satisfied by the attending physician to satisfy the Board of the conditions for involuntary status, the Board declined to make such an order.

By contrast, in *Re LM,* 2007 CanLII 20015 (ON CCB) LM, a 56 year old homeless male with HD had been diagnosed 10 years previously. A psychiatrist gave evidence that LM suffered a disorder secondary to HD or possibly dementia secondary to HD. He was irritable, aggressive, paranoid, on occasions threatening, and displaying cognitive deficits. LM was described as having no insight into his illness or its impact upon him and had repeatedly stated that he was not prepared to take medications. Psychiatric evidence before the Board was that LM lacked the ability to process information relevant to his making decisions about his condition and was unable to appreciate the reasonably foreseeable consequences of his decision-making. The Board concluded that he lacked the capacity to consent to anti-psychotic medication and to benzodiazepines that he required for the treatment of his mental state.

An issue that arises in a number of different contexts in relation to HD is the toll taken by the uncertainty for persons as to whether they will inherit the disease. Deciding whether to have the genetic test to determine whether HD has been inherited can be extremely emotionally fraught. In *Re S,* 2005 CanLII 56704 (ONCCB) S was a 23 year old woman who had been sexually abused by her father and whose mother was murdered by another psychiatric patient when she was 12 years old. She was pregnant and had significant alcohol dependency problems. Her mother and her mother's twin sister had HD but S had declined to ascertain whether she had inherited the condition. She was diagnosed as having paranoid schizophrenia characterized by a range of delusions. The interplay between her self-destructive lifestyle and her anxieties relating to inheriting HD was unclear. The Ontario Care and Consent Board confirmed her involuntary status.

Guardianship Hearings

The most common scenario in which those with HD come into contact with the legal system is when an application is made for a guardian and/or an administrator to be appointed so as to provide for decision-making by others about the person's personal and financial circumstances. Such applications are sometimes welcome and sometimes unwelcome to the patient. On occasions they are contested by the person and/or by some members of the patient's family. Expert evidence by medical practitioners and by social workers is often very important, as are the perspectives of family members and also of the person himself or herself.

In *YW v The Office of the Public Guardian* [2012] ScotSC 114, for instance, Sheriff Lewis dealt with a 37 year old woman with HD, YW, who appealed against a decision of the Public Guardian to grant an application for an access to funds order. She appealed on the basis that the decision was unnecessary as she maintained that she was capable of making decisions in relation to her financial affairs and of safeguarding what she received by way of financial support. She argued that the order that had been made was not the least restrictive option and it was removing from her the last element of control which she had over her life.

Eleven years before she had been diagnosed with HD but by 2012 was presenting with dementia. The Public Guardian maintained that the order in relation to YW was essential as she was mismanaging her financial affairs to such an extent that her physical and mental health were being placed at risk, her standard of living was being seriously compromised and she was vulnerable to exploitation within the community.

Sheriff Lewis found that there was no doubt that the communication skills and mobility of YW were deteriorating. She noted that a support worker had been providing assistance to YW in relation to managing her money beyond the remit of her authority. Sheriff Lewis found that "The appellant has an element of understanding about her condition and of the progressive nature of the disease. She is clearly frustrated not only by the impact of the disease on her life but by what she perceives to be a creeping erosion of her rights and freedoms. That is understandable".

The Sheriff was troubled by the habit of YW in spending "an inordinate proportion of her income on gifts and clothes" for her children: "I am concerned about the immediate capitulation of the appellant to the requests of the children for money or gifts – whether that is attributable to the disease or to a mother's devotion to her children or some other reason I do not know." She noted that YW had a practice of hoarding large sums of money in a handbag that places her in a vulnerable position in the community and at home because she was known locally for her habit. Sheriff Lewis found that YW was increasingly forgetful and that this could lead to the loss of her handbag and its contents, this being the more problematic because YW had "shied away from setting up direct debits or standing orders to pay utilities and rent, preferring to operate a cash based system. She receives a significant amount of money each month by way of benefits yet has left herself so short of money that to pay for food, rent or fuel, she has had to borrow money from her support workers." This led Sheriff Lewis to conclude that YW needed guidance, supervision and support in regard to dealing with daily living expenses and making properly informed choices on spending priorities: "Without that support and guidance, the appellant is simply not capable of looking after her financial affairs." Sheriff Lewis found that intervention would provide a positive benefit for YW: "It will provide certainty in relation to the payment of rent and utilities by way of direct debit or standing order, the regular purchase of food of appropriate quality and quantity, and it will permit a small fund to be built up for the purchase of household appliances. I am of the view that benefit cannot reasonably be achieved without intervention and that form of intervention is the Access to Funds Order." To reduce the extent to which such an order could be counter-therapeutic by depriving YW of all control over her affairs and thereby detracting from her dignity, she allowed her to retain control over some of that income.

In *Re FH* [2005] QGAAT 42, an application was made by a case manager to the Queensland Guardianship and Administration Tribunal for appointment of the Public Trustee of Queensland as administrator over the financial affairs of a 65 year old man, FH, who had HD [38]. He had been admitted shortly previously to hospital after being found paranoid, living in premises that were in disarray and unhygienic – they were also barricaded against entry. FH had a history of alcohol dependence and of setting fires while intoxicated. He had declined home help services. On admission to hospital FH was noted to have cognitive deficits, particularly with regard to orientation and short-term memory – the deficits were consistent with a mild to moderate dementia. He was found to have HD.

FH was described by clinical staff as insightless into his illness and guarded, suspicious and distrustful. Occupational therapy, psychology and social work assessments all recommended supported accommodation for FH. A speech therapy assessment noted early disturbance into his swallowing, a risk factor for his developing aspiration pneumonia. A psychiatrist expressed the view that FH lacked the capacity to make informed decisions regarding personal, health and financial matters. FH was adamant he did not have HD. A neurocognitive assessment showed that FH had significant deficits in visuospatial abilities – he had widespread deficits including frontal network functions such as planning, problem-solving, generation of response alternatives, and the ability to evaluate and modify behaviours: "his adaptive type behaviours were assessed as being so poor that he will experience difficulty in day to day functioning including well-learned tasks." (at [21])

Already he had involuntary movements, restlessness, gait disturbance, poor co-ordination and balance problems.

The Tribunal found that FH was not able to make complex financial decisions and could not understand the nature and effects of decisions about his financial matters, as well as that he had impaired concentration. This meant that in relevant respects he lacked capacity to make financial decisions [39] so it appointed the Public Trustee of Queensland to make financial decisions for FH.

Similarly, in *Re AB* [2008] WASAT 25 the Western Australian State Administrative Tribunal ("the WASAT") was asked by a social worker from an Adult Mental Health Centre to appoint the Public Advocate as limited guardian for a 64 year old woman with HD who was resident in a psychiatric hostel and in a relationship with another hostel resident who informed the WASAT that he and AB intended to marry. She and her partner proposed to leave the hostel and live in a flat which the partner owned. They aspired to receiving assistance from a weekly cleaner and said that they would receive family support. They also planned to travel to visit the family of the partner in the eastern states of Australia and possibly to settle there if the partner obtained employment.

However, the expert evidence was that AB was experiencing significant and increasing difficulties in personal care due to HD and lacked insight into her escalating needs. An Aged Care Assessment Team report noted that AB was displaying short-term memory problems, occasional "at risk" and aggressive behaviours, disturbed sleep, confusion and disorientation. He had been noticed choking on food and required speech therapy assessment. The WASAT concluded that the lack of insight on the part of AB into the effects of her illness potentially placed her at risk "because she requires care and supervision of her medication, her personal hygiene and of her eating because of the risk of choking but does not understand this to be the case" (at [32]). It concluded that AB was unable to make a judgment about her person and because of her disability was in need of oversight, care and control in relation to her health and safety (at [36]). It found that, in spite of AB's expressed wishes and those of her partner, it was in AB's best interests that a guardian be appointed to make decisions in relation to her accommodation, care needs and her travel plans. It appointed the Public Advocate for this function for five years.

The presence of deteriorating symptomatology can be distressing and divisive for the family members of a person diagnosed with HD. In *FE* [2013] WASAT 26 the Western Australian State Administrative Tribunal was asked for a second time to appoint a primary administrator for FE, a woman of 61 with HD diagnosed 10 years previously and associated psychiatric symptomatology. In early 2012 FE had been admitted to hospital with a significant deterioration in her physical and mental health but was discharged after a lengthy period to her home with a service to assist her and monitor her psychiatric medications. Her daughters applied for the appointment of a guardian and administrator because of concerns about their mother being at risk of injury from falls by reason of mobility issues associated with her HD. However, FE's son opposed the making of orders, contending that FE was capable of making her own decisions.

The WASAT made a short-term administration order and adjourned the guardianship application. At the return of the application, medical evidence confirmed underlying brain damage in FE in spite of her having improved somewhat in functioning by reason of treatment. It found that by reason of the disabilities consequent upon brain atrophy FE was not able, because of impaired memory and judgment, to make reasonable decisions regarding her personal or financial affairs, she was not able to look after her own health and safety, and she was in need of oversight and care in the interests of her own health and safety. This meant that she was a person for whom guardianship and administration orders could be made (at [28]). The WASAT found that FE needed assistance with her financial circumstances and because of the progressive nature of her HD appointed an administrator for five years. By the time of the final hearing FE indicated to the WASAT that in spite of opposition from her spouse and her son she believed she needed a guardian to determine the contact she had with family members, including her grandchildren. The WASAT found (at [60]) that informal support from her family had not been sufficient to meet FE's needs in the past, and that it was likely, given the nature of her illness, that her personal needs would increase in the future: "The rejection of professional advice about the represented person needs by her direct carer (the spouse), the conflict within the family about the need for services, and the conflict about the appropriate accommodation for the represented person within the family, which will likely increase as her condition deteriorates, all support the need for a formal order. Because of the statements of the spouse in the final hearing regarding his attitude to his daughters, the Tribunal is not satisfied that the represented person's contact with her daughters and her grandchildren would be maintained without some outside intervention." Accordingly, it appointed an independent statutory official, the Public Advocate, to be FE's guardian for a year with the functions to determine the services to which FE should have access, to make treatment decisions and to determine the contact she would have with family members. It concluded (at [60]) that its order "addresses the immediate needs of the represented person for supervision of her medication, for treatment decisions which take account of her impairments and certainty about contact with her daughters and grandchildren. The longer term need for planning for accommodation into the future can be addressed at the periodic review of the order, or earlier, on application for review, if there is a need."

Family Law

In a variety of circumstances HD can impact upon fitness to parent issues [40] and upon spousal maintenance and division of asset issues. In *S(ER) v S(HC)*, 1998 CanLII 4619 (BCSC), for instance, an application was brought by a husband for division of family assets, spousal maintenance and custody [41]. The wife had HD. Evidence was placed before Levine J from documentation produced by the Huntington Society of Canada, amongst other things observing that "Psychiatric disorders may appear at any time during the course of the disease, even years before motor symptoms develop." (at [7])

Evidence before the Supreme Court of British Columbia was to the effect that the wife was in the middle stages of HD. The husband had custody of their daughter. The division of the spousal assets took account of the fact that he was caring for their child and that the wife required spousal support to pay for her care and living expenses. However, Levine J noted (at [25]) that: "The difficulty is to anticipate her expenses, as they will depend on the progress of her illness." The evidence before the court was that her accommodation was too small, that she needed more care and that she required a companion "to take her on outings, but also for homemaking and personal care. Ultimately, she will require care in a long-term care facility. She is on a waiting list for a government-subsidized room in such a facility." (at [26]) Taking such factors into account, Levine J ordered a division of assets and spousal maintenance and ordered that the husband's obligation to pay spousal support to his wife, should he die before her, would become the obligation of his estate until she passed away.

Another issue that can arise in the family law context is as to whether a court should make an order that children be tested for whether they carry the HD gene. This issue was the subject of an important determination by Baker J in *Re Y and Z (children)* [2013] EWHC 953 (Fam) in respect of male children aged two and three. The father of the children disclosed that his mother and brother suffered from HD and that he suspected he did as as well. The relationship between the children's parents, which had been characterized by drug use and violence, broke down, prompting the local authority to file an application for care orders in respect of the boys. A circuit judge made orders that the boys should be tested for the HD gene and in due course the matter was referred to the Family Division of the High Court of England and Wales.

The local authority supported the testing of the boys and relied on the greatly increased difficulty in finding an adoptive parent for the boys if testing was not undertaken, However, the mother, father and the guardian on behalf of the children all opposed testing, relying on the preponderance of professional opinion on the issue. Concern was also expressed that if one child was found to carry the gene, this could result in the boys being separated by one child being placed for adoption and the other remaining in foster care. In addition, it was argued that there was a likelihood of significant psychological harm for either of the children if they were found to carry the gene.

Justice Baker noted that "it is the general practice not to provide genetic testing to children to determine if they have a condition whise onset occurs in mid adult life where there is no treatment which could be provided in childhood." (at [47]). He also accepted the principle that it is undesirable to treat children differently simply because they are being considered for adoption and concluded that, save in exception al circumstances, children should be given the right to decide for themselves when older whether they should have such a test (at [48]). He acknowledged that adoption might be more difficult if one or both of the children were found to have the gene but did not find this a compelling consideration (at [49]). He gave great importance to the boys being placed permanently together and was concerned at the prospect of their being separated if one of them was found to carry the HD gene (at [50]). Thus, he concluded that it was not in the best interests of the children that the court order that they be genetically tested. The decision is likely to be internationally influential on the issue.

Criminal Law

HD has the potential to affect both criminal responsibility and criminal culpability in significant ways. However, expert evidence that clearly addresses the relevance of the disorder to either criminal responsibility or criminal culpability (at sentencing) is crucial [42].

An early threshold in criminal justice is whether a person is fit to stand trial. Huntington's Disease has the capacity to deprive a person of fitness to participate in the criminal justice process. For instance in *R v Miller*, 2012 BCSC 534 (CanLII) and *R v Miller*, 2011 BCSC 1292 (CanLII) Joyce J of the British Columbia Supreme Court was required on two separate occasions to rule on whether the accused man, who had HD and was charged with murdering his wife, was fit to stand trial. In 2011 his Honour concluded that notwithstanding Miller's cognitive deficits arising from his disease, he could be tried on the basis that in Canada a person only required a "limited cognitive capacity" to understand the process and to communicate with counsel. However, by 2012 the evidence before Joyce J was that Miller's mental state had deteriorated significantly – he had become psychotically delusional with paranoid ideation and very poor memory. He refused to submit to psychological testing and aside from being unable to understand the proceedings against him was assessed as wholly unable to communicate with his counsel. This resulted in him being found on the second occasion to be unfit to stand trial.

In *R v Norman* [2009] EWCA Crim 1810; [2009] Crim LR 346 the appellant, Norman, a 50 year old man, was arrested and charged with child abduction for detaining a child, CM, to keep him out of the lawful control of the child's mother. Norman had been diagnosed in 2003 as suffering from HD. The disease had had a progressive impact upon him. He was examined by three psychiatrists and a clinical neuropsychologist, all of whom concluded that he was not fit to plead and that there was no prospect that he could become so in light of the progressive nature of his illness. Evidence before the trial judge established that Norman had significant vulnerabilities in custody – he had already been subject to "unpleasant treatment" by his fellow prisoners while on remand. In due course he was removed from prison and made the subject of a hospital order after having been found to have committed the offences with which he was charged. However, a crucial aspect to this finding related to the interpretation of a conversation with the child's mother. The Court of Appeal concluded that the jury should have been permitted to hear evidence about the effects of HD on the intentions of the appellant and what he meant in various utterances he made in the course of that conversation. This led to the finding of guilt against him being quashed on appeal.

In *R v Baird* [2002] EWCA 737 the appellant pleaded guilty to causing death by dangerous driving. He contended that at the time of the offence he was suffering depression as a result of his father having been diagnosed with HD and his concern that he too in due course may be affected by the disease.

A psychiatric report suggested that his depression led to a lack of concentration in an otherwise meticulous person and possibly a state of dissociation. A pre-sentence report recommended that sentencing be deferred pending his being tested for HD. However, the sentencing proceeded and he received a sentence of two years' detention in a young offender institution. The Court of Appeal upheld the appeal and substituted a more lenient term of 18 months' detention.

In *R v Larmour* [2004] NICC 4 the effects of HD were considered in a sentencing context. In Northern Ireland At first instance Larmour was sentenced to two terms of life imprisonment for murders he committed in 1987. In 2004 Kerr LCJ and Nicholson LJ heard submissions on the tariff to be set under article 11 of the *Life Sentences (NI) Order 2001* to represent the appropriate sentence for retribution and deterrence before the Life Sentence Review Commissioners could assess his suitability for release on the basis of risk. The killings that he committed were in the company of a loyalist gang associated with the Ulster Freedom Fighters and were premeditated and brutal. However, by 2001 he had been diagnosed as suffering from HD. He was already in need of full-time care and would in due course become increasingly disabled (at [11]). The Crown accepted that his HD could be taken into account in fixing the tariff his sentence. Larmour's HD, along with his youth when he committed the offences, were factored into the decision, resulting in a 15 year tariff being set.

In *R v Jans* [2000] NSWSC 525 the accused pleaded guilty to the manslaughter of his wife whom he stabbed to death with a knife. The evidence was that the prisoner and his wife enjoyed a satisfactory married life of apparently mutual devotion until she commenced to suffer HD. A significant symptom for her was paranoia, characterised by her making multiple accusations against him of infidelity, bisexuality, sexual abuse, trauma and manipulation and by her engaging in multiple acts of physical violence against him. She announced that she intended to seek divorce from him. Unfortunately, for a considerable period of time she was not diagnosed with HD, in part because of her symptoms of breast cancer which resulted in a mastectomy. Justice Grove accepted that Jans' wife's mental state was "a contributing factor in the development of depression in the prisoner. At the time of the killing he was undergoing a major depressive episode" (at [12]). He concluded that the abnormality of mind that Jans suffered was of such a scale and extent as markedly to reduce his level of culpability, resulting in Grove J taking the unusual step of sentencing him only to a four year good behaviour bond for the killing of his wife.

Probate

The capacity of a person with HD to make a will – to have testamentary capacity – can be complex [43]. In addition, there can be difficult issues in relation to the needs of a person with HD after the death of a spouse or partner. In *Gully v Dix* [2004] EWCA Civ 139; [2004] 1 WLR 1399 Mrs Gully had left her husband to live with the deceased in 1974 but they never married although they lived in a bona fide marriage-like relationship. However, the deceased became addicted to alcohol which led to multiple separations between the parties and an attempt on his part to commit suicide, after which Mrs Gully looked after him in conditions that were increasingly squalid. Her difficulties were compounded by her being diagnosed in 1991 with HD. In 2001 he separated from Mrs Gully after he attacked her in the night with a knife. The separation was short-lived as he was found dead in his garden some three months later.

This led to an inquiry into whether at the time of his death the deceased was living in his household with Mrs Gully for the purposes on the *Inheritance (Provision for Family and Dependents Act) 1975* (UK). The Court of Appeal found that "the steadfastness of a commitment to live together may wax and wane, but so long as it is not extinguished, it survives."(at [24]) This permitted the claim by Mrs Gully. What was not canvassed was the extent of Mrs Gully's needs in light of her having becoming symptomatic with HD.

Compensation

Whether a person previous to a tortious event had or later developed HD [44] can impact upon damages awarded given that while it is orthodox law that the tortfeasor takes their victim as they find them, they are also generally only responsible for the harm that they cause. Thus in *Hefferland v Fink*, 1995 CanLII 2047 (BC SC) at [30] MacKinnon J of the Supreme Court of British Columbia found that a compensable accident sustained by the plaintiff "has compounded and aggravated the problems he had with Huntington's Disease. His walking is now extremely slow and awkward. Now his speech is such that it is difficult to comprehend him. He is now unable to swim. He now has no sexual relations and doesn't expect he will in the future."

In *Kakoschke v Draper* [2006] QSC 386 the plaintiff, a woman of 43, suffered injuries in a motor vehicle collision. The physical sequelae from the collision were minor and the basis for the plaintiff's economic loss claim was a contention that she suffered from a psychiatric illness brought on by the collision. A complicating factor was that she had been sexually abused as a child by her grandfather. She also carried the gene for HD and was either symptomatic or in due course would become so. Psychiatric opinions about her condition varied. One expert expressed the view that the plaintiff had PTSD. Another said she did not. One psychiatrist opined that her knowledge that she was carrying the HD gene was causing depression, including at the time of the accident. A neurologist expressed the view that she was showing mild choreiform movements and that "her recent development of mood changes, depression and anxiety, probably represents the early stages of Huntington's disease." (at [36]). Skoien AJ did not accept this latter view on the basis of there not being sufficient evidence to support it.

The plaintiff was assessed by Queensland Health as a person able to cope with learning that she was a carrier of the gene after her family learned that her father had HD. In 2003 she learned that she too carried the gene and had a "repeat count" of 43, much the same as the count of 42 of her father with diagnosed HD. Skoien AJ commented that: "The 'repeat count' indicates the abnormality which, if it exceeds 37 means that the carrier will contract the disease. Her increased repeat count is minor, considering it may be measured in the 80's or higher." (at [32]).

Ultimately Skoien AJ accepted that the only cause of the plaintiff's serious psychiatric disability was the motor vehicle accident [45]. However, Skoien AJ also needed to consider its relevance in terms of being a supervening factor in her ability to return to work. He noted that the "early manifestations of HD "may include difficulty in co-ordination, involuntary movements, difficulty in planning and often a depressed or irritable mood." (at [30]) He observed that the plaintiff's father suffered the onset of HD to a noticeable degree probably when he was in his mid-60s. He concluded that it was likely that the plaintiff would contract HD at a similar stage to that of her father or perhaps a little earlier given that she already had a slightly increased repeat count. In turn, this impacted to some degree upon the assessment of the damages to be awarded.

Conclusion

HD is a profoundly confronting condition. Once its symptoms manifest, it is relentlessly progressive. The prospect of its symptomatology is frightening and extremely stressful for those who either know they have the Hungtington's gene or who know that family members have or have had the disease. HD affects both the mind and the body in inexorable and devastating ways. As the International Huntington Association puts it, "HD is a family disease because of its impact on every family member [46]". Finding perspective in relation to HD is difficult; not everyone reaches the point of Barema [47]: "It all depends on your angle, your take on life. Because eventually, we are all going to come apart. We'll all go through it. Yes, we've all got some Huntington's in us." Not surprisingly, HD is accompanied by high levels of depression and suicidality in the anticipatory, prodromal and symptomatic phases.

In the legal context HD has multiple repercussions of which it is constructive for those with the condition, those at risk of the condition, and those caring for those with the condition, to be conscious. It can result in unfairly stigmatizing discrimination in workplace and insurance contexts. It can also result in unfitness to give evidence [48], unfitness to make decisions as a litigant and unfitness to stand trial. A consequence of HD symptomatology at some point is increasingly impaired capacity in multiple other areas as well, including capacity to make decisions in the context of involuntary inpatient or outpatient status, the need for a guardian or administrator, and capacity to exercise testamentary capacity. Awareness of these legal consequences of the disease emphasizes the need for encouragement by medical and legal personnel toward forward planning (by adults) , while it is still possible, for those with HD so that as much leeway as possible can be extended by advance directives and other means of communication on the part of the person with the disease. In this way, they can take as much control for as long as possible in relation to their lives and the management of their condition.

HD can eliminate criminal responsibility and reduce criminal culpability, but this depends on the extent of symptomatology at the time of commission of criminal offences and at the time of sentencing. Courts are dependent in this regard upon well focused and argued expert reports (and oral testimony) from health practitioners, often those who are treating the accused person.

The special needs of a person with HD can impact upon their entitlement to damages arising out of a tortious incident and can increase their need for special provision under spousal maintenance obligations in family law, and their own ability to pay child support or spousal maintenance. They can also be relevant in the context of testator's family maintenance claims.

The decided cases reveal the difficulty of identifying with clarity the status of a person's HD symptomatology at any given time, especially when alternative aetiologies exist for symptoms experienced by a patient, including when the symptoms are principally affective.

An issue which has arisen in the course of litigation has been the impact of a person experiencing stress in relation to HD - whether it is as to the potential for their developing HD or whether they may have transmitted it to a child or grandchild. Many persons do not wish definitive diagnosis but ongoing potential to be HD-positive can wreak its own damage and can be very difficult to live with. This can result in lifestyle decisions that are reckless and risky [49]. In addition, living with a person with HD can be exceptionally problematic because of the risk of paranoid, violent and disordered ideation at some stage on the part of the person with HD. This in itself can be psychogenic and criminogenic, as well as corrosive on the wellbeing of loved ones; the disorder has secondary victims too. Even survivor guilt for those who do not inherit HD can have its own difficulties [50]. Care needs to be taken in imposing upon persons at risk of the condition knowledge that they have the HD gene, especially when they are children.

However, there are elements to the HD experience that have little to do with the law but from which lawyers and clinicians alike can learn. After all, a person is not their disease. All is not entirely negative in relation to the disease. As a wife of a middle-aged man with HD [52] has said, after emphasizing the grim realities of HD: "Being able to live in the moment is Huntington's greatest gift. ... After you've finished grieving for your lost future (which can take years), you realize that the imagined future you are grieving for was never real anyway. Huntington's shocks you into an appreciation that all we have, really, is 'now'. Your plans, even your subconscious ones, aren't your life. Moments are your life."

References

[1] Compare Sydenham's chorea, also known as Chorea minor or St Vitus' dance: see Waller J, *A Time to Dance, A Time to Die* (Icon Books, Cambridge, 2008); Hannah P, "Huntington's Chorea or Sydenham's Chorea: Two Major Forms of Chorea" (23 March 2013):

http://www.associatedcontent.com/article/2354268/huntingtons_chorea_and_sydenhams_chorea.html, viewed 29 March 2013.

[2] Wexler A, *The Woman Who Walked into the* Sea (Yale University Press, New Haven, 2008), at p174ff. See too in relation to sterilisation of persons with, amongst other things, HD pursuant to the *Sexual Sterilization Act*, SA,1928, *Muir v Alberta* (1996) 132 DLR (4th) 695.

[3] See discussion in *Soulitopoulos v LaTrobe University Liberal Club* [2002] FCA 1316 at [35]-[38]; Wexler A, *The Woman Who Walked into the* Sea (Yale University Press, New Haven, 2008), at p175. See further Lifton RJ, *The Nazi Doctors: Medical Killing and the Psychology of* Genocide (Basic Books, New York, 1986); Freckelton I, "Bioethics, Biopolitics and Medical Regulation: Learning from the Nazi Doctor Experience" (2009) 16 JLM 555.

[4] http://frank.mtsu.edu/~baustin/nurmlaw1.html , viewed 10 March 2013.

[5] See *Huntington's Disease Parity Act 2013* (US): HR 1015.

[6] See Australian Law Reform Commission, *Essentially Yours: The Protection of Human genetic Information* (ALRC 96, AGPS, Canberra, 2003): http://www.austlii.edu.au/au/other/alrc/publications/reports/96/, viewed 30 March 2013; Williams JK et al, "In their own Words: Reports of Stigma and Genetic Discrimination by People at Risk for Huntington Disease in the International RESPOND-HD Study" (2010) 153B (6) Am J Med Genet B Neuropsychiatr Genet 1150-1159; Kirby M, "Human Genome Project: Legal Issues", paper to Australian Lawyers' Conference, Hanoi, Vietnam, 10 July 1999: http://www.hcourt.gov.au/assets/publications/speeches/former-justices/kirbyj/kirbyj_humang.htm, viewed 29 March 2013; Jensen P, "Genetic Privacy: The Potential for Genetic Discrimination in Insurance" (1999) 33*Victoria University of Wellington Law Review* 379.

[7] See Knowles J, *Huntington's Disease* (Rosen Publishing, New York, 2006).

[8] Huntingtons Outreach Project for Education at Stanford, "Protein Aggregation": http://www.stanford.edu/group/hopes/cgi-bin/wordpress/2011/06/about-protein-aggregation/, viewed 29 March 2013.

[9] Gharibzadeh et al have argued that glutamate toxicity is the cause of HD: see Gharibzadeh S, Sarbaz, Y, Banaie M and Towhidshah F, "Two Novel Comments on the Treatment of Huntington's Disease" (2009) 21 *Journal of Clinical Neuropsychiatry and Clinical Neurosciences* 98.

[10] See Monche-Buchner E et al, "Counting CAG Repeats in the Huntington's Disease Gene by Restriction Endonuclease *Eco*P15I

Cleavage" (2002) 30(16) *Nucleic Acids Research* e83. See too National Human Genome Research Institute, "Learning about Huntington's Disease": http://www.genome.gov/10001215, viewed 29 March 2013.

[11] Better Health, "Huntington's Disease – Genetics": http://www.betterhealth.vic.gov.au/bhcv2/bhcarticles.nsf/pages/Huntingtons_disease_genetics?open, viewed 29 March 2013.

[12] The structure in the forebrain whose main function is to regulate movement and influence various types of learning, utilizing dopamine.

[13] Revilla FJ and Grutzendler J, "Huntington Disease" (4 September 2008): http://emedicine.medscape.com/article/1150165-overview, viewed 29 March 2013.

[14] See Folstein SE, *Huntington's Disease: A Disorder of Families* (The Johns Hopkins University Press, Boston,1989).

[15] McCarthy DJ, Alexander R, Smith MA, Pathak S, Kanes S, Lee CM, and Sanacora G, "Glutamate-based Depression GBD" (2012) 78(5) Med Hypotheses 675-681.

[16] Quarrell O, *Huntington's Disease* , 2nd edn (Oxford University Press, Oxford, 2008), at p28

[17] Halpin M, "Accounts of Suicidality in the Huntington Disease Community" (2012) 65(4) Omega (Westport) 317-334.

[18] Epping EA and Paulsen JS, "Depression in the Early Stages of Huntington Disease" (2011) 1(5) Neurodegener Dis Manag.407-414.

[19] Wetzel HH, Gehl CR, Dellefave-Castillo L, Schiffman JF, Shannon KM, and Paulsen JS; "Suicidal Ideation in Huntington Disease: the Role of Comorbidity" (2011) 188(3) Psychiatry Res 372-6. See too Hubers AA, Reedeker N, Giltay EJ, Roos RA, van Duijn E, and van der Mast RC. "Suicidality in Huntington's Disease" (2012) 136(3) J Affect Disord. 550-557.

[20] Quarrell, at p7.

[21] *See Carter v Canada (Attorney General),* 2012 BCSC 886 (CanLII) at [1041].

[22] Adema S, Jansen I, van Zwol E, "Euthanasia in Huntington's Disease Patients in the Netherlands: a Reconnaissance" (2010) *J Neurol Neurosurg Psychiatry* 2010;81:A45 doi.

[23] National Institute of Neurological Disorders and Stroke, *Huntington's Disease Information Page*: http://www.ninds.nih.gov/disorders/huntington/huntington.htm, viewed 29 March 2013.

[24] See Quarrell OWJ, *Juvenile Huntington's Disease And Other Trinucleotide Repeat Disorders* (Oxford University Press, Melbourne, 2009).

[25] Nance M, Jones R, Imriglio S and Gettig B, Juvenile Huntington's Disease (Huntington's Disease Society of America, New York): http://www.huntington-assoc.com/Juv._HD.pdf, viewed 29 March 2013

[26] Family Caregiver Alliance, "Huntington's Disease" http://www.caregiver.org/caregiver/jsp/content_node.jsp?nodeid=574, viewed 29 March 2013.

[27] National Human Genome Research Institute, "Learning about Huntington's Disease": http://www.genome.gov/10001215, viewed 28 March 2013.

[28] Quarrell O, *Huntington's Disease* , 2nd edn (Oxford University Press, Oxford, 2008), at p5.

[29] However, overall in Australia HD is said by Huntingtons Australia to affect six to seven people in every 100,000: Huntingtons Australia: http://huntingtonsaustralia.asn.au/, viewed 28 March 2013.

[30] FJ Revilla and J Grutzendler, "Huntington Disease" (4 September 2008): http://emedicine.medscape.com/article/1150165-overview, viewed 28 March 2013.

[31] Wild EJ and Tabrizi SJ, "Differential Diagnosis of Chorea" (2007) 7 Pract Neurol 360 at 362-363.

[32] See Huntington's Disease Society of America, "Genetics and Genetic Testing": http://www.hdsa.org/living-with-huntingtons/publications/index.html#ggt, viewed 28 March 2013.

[33] See Rohs G and Klimek ML, "Ethical, Social and Legal Issues in Huntington Disease: The Nurse's Role" (1996) 17(3) *Axone* 55-59; CL Becker, "Legal Implications of the G-8 Huntington's Disease Genetic Marker" (1989) 39 *Case Western Reserve Law Review* 273.

[34] See Terrenoire G, "Huntington's Disease and the Ethics of Genetic Prediction" (1992) 18(2) *Journal of Medical Ethics* 79-85; B Steinbock and R McClamrock, "When Is Birth Unfair to the Child?" Hastings Center Report: http://www.albany.edu/~ron/papers/badbirth.html, viewed 23 March 2013; Huggins M, Bloch M, Kanani S, Quarrell OW, Theilman J, Hedrick A, Dickens B, Lynch A, and Hayden M, "Ethical and Legal Dilemmas Arising during *Predictive Testing for Adult-onset Disease*: The Experience of Huntington Disease" (1990) 47(1) American Journal of Human Genetics 4–12.

[35] See eg Okinata N, "Genetic Screening and Insurance: Too Valuable an Underwriting Tool to be Banned from the System" (1992) 98(1) *Santa Clara Computer and High Technology Law Journal* 145-167.

[36] Huntington's Disease Association, "Huntington's Disease and the Law": http://hda.org.uk/hda/factsheets, viewed 23 March 2013.

[37] Oster E, Dorsey ER, Bausch J, Shinaman A, Elise Kayson E, Oakes D, Shoulson I, Quaid K, "Fear of Health Insurance Loss among Individuals at Risk for Huntington Disease" (2008) 146A *American Journal of Medical Genetics* 2070-2077.

[38] See too *Ps and Ss* [2005] WASAT 231; *Re WSF* [2006] QGAAT 79; Re HVM [2006] QGAAT 37; *Re WAB* [2007] QGAAT 12; *Re PAC* [2007] QGAAT 54.

[39] Under Schedule 4 of the *Guardianship and Administration Act 2000* (Qld) he lacked capacity.

[40] See eg the arguments raised in *KM v GEM*, 2005 ABQB 651.

[41] See too *Jenkins v Repatriation Commission* [1999] FCA 269.

[42] Compare *R v Belcourt*, 2000 BCAA 441 (CanLII).

[43] See *In The Estate of Stefan Miegoch No. 119295/93 Wills - Solicitors* [1996] NSWSC 68.

[44] See eg *Hefferland v Fink*, 1995 CanLII 2047 (BC SC) where the plaintiff in an action for damages arising from a motor car accident had HD and the court found (at [30]) that "The accident has compounded and aggravated the problems he had with Huntington's Disease. His walking is now extremely slow and awkward. Now his speech is such that it is difficult to comprehend him. He is now unable to swim. He now has no sexual relations and doesn't expect he will in the future." See also *Forbes v Quinn* [2011] NIQB 14.

[45] See the similar issue which arose in a different compensation context in *Hales and Repatriation Commission* [2003] AATA 530.

[46] International Huntington Association" http://www.huntington-assoc.com/, viewed 6 July 2010.

[47] Barema J, *The Test: Living in the Shadow of Huntington's Disease* (Franklin Square Press, New York, 2005), at p160.

[48] *Caddy v Mcinnes* [1995] FCA 1464; (1995) 131 ALR 277; see too *Langridge v Nifort*, 1991 CanLII 4477 (NSSC)

[49] See eg *Re S*, 2005 CanLII 56704 (ON CCB).

[50] See Stauffer J, "Dealing with Survivor Guilt" (2010) 109 *Huntington's News* 3: http://www.huntingtons.org.nz/news_109.pdf, viewed 20 July 2010.

[51] See Sulaiman S, *Learning to Live with Huntington's Disease: One Family's Story* (Jessica Kingsley Publishers, London, 2007), at p132-133.

Index

D

E

F

G

H

I

O

P

T

U

V

W

Y